Essential Skills

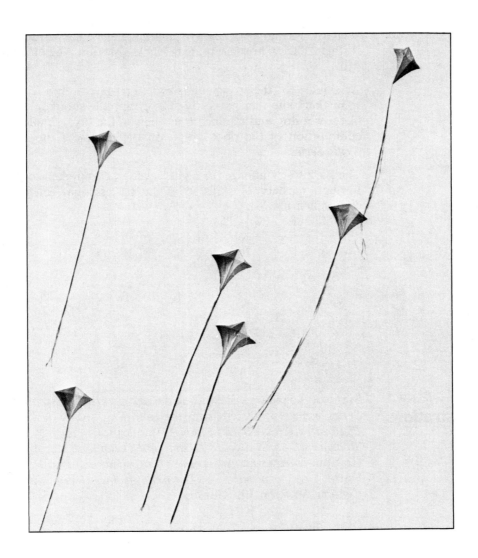

Revised Edition

About the Cover

The breeze was fresh this bright day in May, and gaily-colored kites appeared like spring swallows, darting across the blue sky over Rhode Island's Narragansett Bay. Photographer Tony Botelho was there to capture on film the kite-flights of Christy Menard, Art Pelosi, Danny Champagne, Peggy Hulsey, John Rathjen, Jack Christie, Stephen Jencks, Marion Alig and Megen Mills.

A salute to the rowboaters who retrieved the "diamond-spinnaker" kite that got away! The errant kite shook in the wind like a wet dog and rejoined the others in the sky, completing the composition of the photograph on the covers of the *Essential Skills Series*.

The six kites symbolize the higher levels of comprehension gained through mastery of skills from the six essential categories of comprehension.

About the Illustrations

Many of the pictures illustrating the passages in the *Essential Skills Series* were reproduced from the following books in the *Dover Pictorial Archive Series*, Dover Publications, Inc., New York: *Treasury of Art Nouveau, Design and Ornament*, Carol Belanger Grafton; *Harter's Picture Archive for Collage and Illustration*, Jim Harter; and *Animals: A Pictorial Archive from Nineteenth-Century Sources*, Jim Harter.

Other illustrations are by Howard Lewis and Thomas Ewing Malloy.

Essential Skills Series

Essential Skills Book 6

Walter Pauk, Ph.D.
Director, Reading Research Center
Cornell University

Revised Edition

Jamestown Publishers
Providence, Rhode Island

Essential Skills Series
No. 306, Book 6

Copyright © 1982 by Jamestown Publishers, Inc.

All rights reserved. The contents of this book are protected by the United States Copyright Law. It is illegal to copy or reproduce any pages or parts of any pages. Address all inquiries to Editor, Jamestown Publishers, Post Office Box 9168, Providence, Rhode Island 02940.

Cover Design by Deborah Hulsey Christie, adapted from the Original Design by Stephen R. Anthony

Text Design by Deborah Hulsey Christie

Printed in the United States AL

88 89 90 91 92 11 10 9 8 7 6

ISBN 0-89061-225-0

Preface

Practice Makes Perfect

Why do some students shoot baskets over and over again and others skate and reskate the same routine? These beginners know that practice makes perfect. Not only do beginners know this, but pros do too. For what other reason do they work at baseball and football week after week before the opening dates?

Value of Practice

The pros know the value of practice, but they also know the value of something else. They know that practice without *instruction* and *guidance* does not automatically lead to improvement. That's why they have the best coaches that money can buy.

And so it is with developing the skills of reading. There must be the right kind of practicing and the right kind of coaching.

First, a word about practice. In this book the right kind of practice is provided by twenty-five highly interesting and carefully selected passages. Here is material enough on which to grow and keep growing.

Value of Coaching

Now about coaching! Good coaching takes the form of instruction and guidance. In this book the instruction is straightforward and uncomplicated. It puts you directly on the right track, and better still, you are kept on the right track by two unusual systems of guidance. The first system is the uniquely designed, six-way question format which makes sure that every ounce of practice is directed toward improvement. Nothing is wasted!

Diagnostic Chart

The second system of guidance is the Diagnostic Chart. This chart is no ordinary gimmick. In truth, it provides the most dignified form of diagnosis and guidance yet devised. It provides instantaneous and continuous diagnosis and gentle but certain self-guidance. It yields information directly to the student. This form of self-guidance leads to the goal of all education: the goal of self-teaching.

Acknowledgments

Now, I want to make some acknowledgments, especially to the students who were the guinea pigs. Afterwards I told them so, but they said, "We didn't mind even then. And now that it is over, we're all the happier because we know how much we've learned." But what the students did not know was how much I learned from them. For this I thank them all, class after class.

I direct especial thanks to Linda Browning, Anita DuBose, and Karen Duddy for handling the almost countless number of selections, writing and refining the questions and making sure that the series kept moving: all, a most demanding task.

Finally, I am most grateful to authors, editors and publishers who have generously given permission to quote and reprint in this book from works written and published by them. The books quoted in the text and used as sources of reading extracts are listed in the back of the book.

Walter Pauk

Contents

To the Instructor **8**

To the Student **11**

    Understanding the Six Essential Skills **11**
    Answering the Main Idea Question **17**
    Getting the Most Out of This Book **19**

Passages and Questions **23**

Answer Key **100**

Diagnostic Chart **102**

Progress Graph **103**

Classroom Management System **106**

To the Instructor

Selection of Passages

All of us believe in this truism: to learn to read, a person must read. But, placing a book in front of a student won't automatically promote reading.

This last sentence brings up another truism: you can lead a horse to water, but you can't make it drink. To tempt a horse, the water must be clear, cool and clean.

To tempt the student, the passages must be genuinely fascinating. Knowing this, we packed each book with twenty-five "I can't put the book down" type of passages.

Each passage had to meet at least the following criteria: *high interest level, appropriate readability level* and *factual accuracy of contents*. High interest was assured by choosing passages from popular magazines that appeal to a wide range of readers. The readability level of each passage was assessed by applying Dr. Edward B. Fry's *Formula for Estimating Readability,* thus enabling the arrangement of passages on a single grade level within each book. The factual accuracy of the passages is high because they were written by professional writers whose works are recognized and respected.

The Great Value of Questions

Dr. Mortimer J. Adler says that the overall secret for improving one's reading can be boiled down to knowing how to keep awake while reading. He means more than keeping one's eyes open. He means keeping one's mind open and active.

One sure-fire way to do this is to keep trying to answer questions while reading. Questions not only keep one's mind awake, but also keep the mind active, not letting it get flabby. Here's a good story that makes the same point.

> To keep their fish alive for the fresh-fish markets, the owners of fishing boats used a water-filled floating tank. The fish remained alive all right, but they were never firm, always flabby. One captain, however, always brought back firm, fresh, active fish. His fish always received a higher price.

One day he revealed his secret: "You see," he said, "for every hundred herrings I put into my tank, I put in one catfish. It is true that the catfish eat five or six of the herrings on the trip back to port, but the catfish keep the rest alert and constantly active. That's why my herring arrive in beautiful condition."

The work of the catfish, in this book, is done by the six essential questions (subject matter, supporting details, conclusion, clarifying devices, vocabulary in context, and main idea). These questions keep the minds of students alert, active and in beautiful condition.

The main idea questions in this book are not the usual multiple-choice variety. Given four statements, the students are asked to recognize the main idea of the passage. They also tell why each of the other three does not express the main idea; the students identify one statement as too narrow, one as too broad and one as merely a detail.

By asking these six types of questions in each passage, students quickly learn to read with a questioning and anticipating attitude. This attitude, necessary for high comprehension, is easily transferred to other material such as the textbook.

The Diagnostic Chart

Those who used the first edition of these books had high praise for the Diagnostic Chart. In sum, this is what they said.

> The Diagnostic Chart is truly ingenious because it is, in fact, a self-diagnosing instrument. The Chart instantly, simply and continually shows students their strengths and weaknesses.

Here is how the Chart works. The six questions for each passage are always in the same order. For example, the question designed to teach the skill of making *conclusions* is always in the number three position, and the question designed to teach the skill of identifying *clarifying devices* is always in the number four position, and so forth. This innovation of keeping the questions in order sets the stage for the smooth functioning of the Chart.

The Chart works automatically when the letters of the answers are placed in the spaces on the Chart. Even after completing one passage, the Chart will reveal the type or types of questions answered correctly as well as the types answered incorrectly. But more important, the Chart will identify the types of questions missed consistently. More persuasive identification is possible after three or more passages have been completed. By then, a pattern can be observed. For example, if the answers to question number three (making conclusions) are incorrect for all three passages, or on three out of four, then this weakness shows up automatically.

Once a weakness is revealed, instruct the students to take the following steps: First, turn back to the instructional pages to study the section in which the topic is discussed. Second, go back to read again the questions in that particular category that were missed; then, with the correct answers in mind, read the entire passage again, trying to see how the author developed the answers to the questions. Third, on succeeding passages, put forth extra effort to answer correctly the questions in that particular category. Fourth, if the difficulty still persists, arrange for a conference with the instructor.

To the Student

Understanding the Six Essential Skills

How do readers get the meaning from written words? To get meaning, readers need to know at least six essential skills.

1. Subject Matter — Readers need to know how to concentrate or focus on the writing. This helps them learn what the writing is about.
2. Main Idea — Readers need to know how to grasp the main idea or point of the writing.
3. Supporting Details — Readers need to be able to connect supporting details to the ideas.
4. Conclusions — Readers should be able to come to conclusions or guess endings based on the ideas.
5. Clarifying Devices — Readers should be able to note the writer's methods of making the points clear and alive.
6. Vocabulary in Context — Readers must know what the words in the writing mean.

Let's take a closer look at these six skills.

Concentration/Subject Matter

One thing readers often say is, "I can't concentrate!" But there is a sure, fast cure. There is no better way to gain concentration when reading than this. Read the first few lines. Then ask yourself these questions: "What is this passage about?" "What is the subject matter?"

If you don't ask these questions, here's what may happen. Your eyes will move across the lines of print. Yet your mind will be thinking of other things.

But if you ask the questions, you will most likely get an answer, thus achieving concentration. Let's see if this method works. Here are the first lines of a passage:

> Wood ducks are the most beautiful ducks in North America. Once they were rare. Now — if you have sharp eyes and can keep quiet — you might see them in almost any woodland along streams and ponds.

After reading this, you can see that the author will talk about the wood duck. Now that your mind is on the trail, the chances are good it will follow the author's idea line by line. Thus, you will *concentrate* on the building of the subject matter.

Let's try the method again. Here are a few lines from another passage:

> Of all the little animals in the world, the Columbian ground squirrel is one of the liveliest and friendliest. It is nicknamed "picket pin." This is because it sits as stiff and straight as a stake in the ground.

Again, you most likely had no trouble picking out the subject. It is the Columbian ground squirrel.

Main Idea Once the subject matter has been grasped, it is time for the next question. Ask yourself, "What is the author's main idea?" "What point is the passage trying to make?"

With such questions in mind, you can be sure an answer will often pop up. But when no questions are asked, all things seem the same. Nothing stands out. The reader will not see the point of the passage.

Let's look at another passage. This time we will find the main idea.

> Wood ducks never nest on the ground as most ducks do, but in a big hole in a tree. Trees with big holes in them are hard to find.

You don't have the full passage to read, so I will tell you the answer. The main point is that with fewer and fewer old, dead trees with big holes in them, we will have fewer and fewer wood ducks.

Thus, when questions are asked, the reader is acting upon the content. Reading becomes a two-way street with both reader and writer engaged. In a sense, the reader talks with the author. So the passage comes to life. Reading then is a joy.

Supporting Details

Do we like details? Of course we do. In long pieces of writing, main ideas are like the bones. They are the skeleton of the writing. The details are the flesh. They give the writing fullness and life.

Details are used to support the main ideas. So the term *supporting details* fits well. These supporting details come in many forms. The most common forms are examples, definitions, comparisons, contrasts, repetitions and descriptions.

The author of "The Wood Duck" lets us know that the passage is about wood ducks. Next, the author makes sure we learn that the point is that without trees with holes, the wood duck will not nest. Thus, there would be fewer wood ducks.

Now that we are involved in this problem, the author gives us details on how we can provide trees with holes in them. The author *describes* how we can build a wood duck nesting box. Here's the excerpt:

> Why don't you and your parents put up a wood duck nesting box right now? It would be about two feet (about .61 meters) high and ten inches (about 25.4 centimeters) square. Make the entry hole about four inches (about 10.2 centimeters) across. Use rough lumber on the inside, so the ducklings can climb up the sides to the hole. Put wood shavings on the bottom. In these the duck will lay her eggs. To keep her eggs warm, she covers them with her own feathers. If you can't find a tree near the water, you will need a post. Place the box ten to thirty feet (about 3.1 to 9.1 meters) high.

You can see in the above passage how important details are in telling a story. Details let the reader see what's going on. They paint a vivid picture of the action. They may tell how to do something. They may tell how something happened.

In long passages there will also be sub-ideas. It is important to be careful not to mistake a sub-idea for a main idea. Sub-ideas are broader than details. But sub-ideas are still not the main point. The main idea has to do with the whole passage. The sub-idea has to do with just part of it. Note that in the next sample, the sub-idea is about the food that wood ducks eat. The whole passage is not about food. Thus, food is *not* the main idea. For the most part, you will see that a sub-idea takes the space of one paragraph. Often, the topic sentence of the paragraph is a statement of a sub-idea.

The following excerpts show how the author groups and structures supporting details around the sub-ideas that are stated in topic sentences. A sub-idea will hold a group of details together.

> Wood ducks eat acorns and all kinds of nuts. Their stomachs (or gizzards) have strong muscles. They can break the hardest nuts, some that you could barely crack with a hammer, in their stomachs. Wood ducks like berries, duckweed and insects. But best of all they like to eat spiders. That's ice cream to them.

The topic sentence is the first sentence. It states that the sub-idea is the foods wood ducks eat. Next, the author describes how the newly hatched ducklings get down to the ground from the nest.

Here are more details grouped around a sub-idea.

> Sometimes they nest in holes up in trees that are twice as high as a flagpole. Just think, the baby ducklings must jump to the ground the day they hatch. They don't get hurt, though, because they're light, like little puffs of cotton. The mother stands at the foot of the tree and calls and calls. The ducklings peek out of the hole. Then, like little paratroopers, they jump quickly, one right after the other, to join their mother. She must then hurry them to the pond where they're safe.

Thus, one of the main jobs of *supporting details* is to give some fullness to the passage. The passage would be just a boring, skimpy statement of the main idea with its bare-boned sub-ideas if not for details. The details give the passage life.

Conclusion The reader will move through a passage, grasping the main and sub-ideas and their details. It is then common for the reader to start to guess a conclusion or ending to the story. Such guesses are part of the sport of reading. Often, the author gives the reader an ending. In such a case, the joy of reading lies in the fact that the reader finds out the guess was right. But the ending may not be given. The reader then will try to guess the ending that is hinted by the author.

The conclusion from the excerpts just read about the wood duck is in having the reader see the pleasure of observing a wood duck. The final sentence is this:

> If you're lucky, though, and if your (duck) house is in place before the ice melts, you will have a wood duck family in the summer.

In a passage called "From Pond to Prairie," the author has this conclusion:

> Finally, there is no longer much open water. The pond has disappeared. Depending on the kinds of plants that have filled it, the pond may be called a bog or a marsh. As changes continue for many more years, the bog may become a forest.

The skillful reader is like a detective. This reader follows the story, always thinking, "Where is the author leading me?" "What's the final point?" "What's the conclusion?" And the reader, like a detective, must try to guess the conclusion, changing the guess if necessary as the story unfolds.

Clarifying Devices The author uses clarifying devices to make the points in the story clear and alive. In a sense, the *topic sentence* may be thought of as a clarifying device. It is often placed at the start of a paragraph. In this way, the author gives the reader a quick point of focus.

The point of the passage becomes clear after reading it.

But more often, by clarifying devices, we mean the literary devices in the passage. These are words or phrases which keep the ideas, sub-ideas and details in clear focus and in order.

Authors use literary devices to make details clear and interesting. An example of a device is the *metaphor,* as in "But best of all they like to eat spiders. *That's ice cream to them.*"

One more literary device is the *simile.* "*Like little paratroopers,* they (the ducklings) jump quickly, one right after the other, to join their mother," is a simile. The simile helps the reader imagine a vivid scene. It brings to the mind of the reader something known — paratroopers. Then it compares the known idea to the ducklings' jump from their nest to make a fresh, new idea. It is fun to imagine the little ducks copying real paratroopers jumping from a plane.

Besides metaphors and similes, other *clarifying devices* are organizational patterns. One common pattern is to unfold the events in the order of time. Thus, one thing happens first and then another and another, and so forth.

The time pattern orders the event. The event may take place in the span of five minutes. It may last hundreds of years. A time pattern may be used to relate the habits of an animal from its birth to its death.

You should learn to find these literary devices. They help you to understand the passage and speed your reading.

Vocabulary in Context

A reader who does not know what the author's words mean may not understand the passage. A reader should look up in the dictionary the unknown words.

Also a reader may understand only the general meaning of the word. But sometimes a more *exact* meaning is needed to grasp the passage fully. A reader who places a general meaning on a word may end up with a blurred picture of the idea. An exact meaning will give the reader a full and clear picture.

For instance, in the next excerpt are two common words that many people feel they already know. Thus, they don't see the need to look them up in the dictionary. But few people know the exact meaning of these words.

> Depending on the kinds of plants that have filled it, the pond may be called a *bog* or a *marsh*.

Do you know the difference between a bog and a marsh? Is there a difference? If so, what is it? How would your mental picture change if you knew?

Looking up words for their exact meanings is rewarding. A precise vocabulary leads to true understanding.

You may find it troublesome to look up words you feel you already know. But you should get into this habit to improve your reading. Of course, words you do not know must always be looked up. You would most likely need a dictionary for these words:

> Nothing could appear more *benign* than a field aglow with daisies, goldenrod and Queen Anne's lace.
>
> *Sphinxlike,* it crouches among the flowers until the desired insect wanders within reach.

The dictionary is like a stock market. Here you exchange fuzzy meanings for exact meanings. You get new meanings for unknown words. All this is at no cost. It takes just a flip of your finger.

Answering the Main Idea Question

To be able to find the main idea of the things you read is important. It is one of the best reading skills you can learn. The main idea questions in this book are not the ones you've seen where you pick just the right answer. Instead, each main idea question is made up of four statements. Two of the statements refer to just parts of the passage. One of these is a *detail*. It states a point. But that point has little to do with the passage as a whole. The next statement is *too narrow*. It tells more than the detail statement. Still, it's too specific to tell about the main point of the passage. The "too narrow" statement is often a sub-idea.

The last two statements deal with the whole passage. One is *too broad*. It is too general and too vague to be a good main idea statement. The final statement is the *main idea*. It tells *who* or *what* the point of the passage is. The main idea statement answers the question *does what?* or *is what?* also.

Read the sample passage below. Then follow the instructions in the box. The answer to each part of the main idea question has been filled in for you. The score for each answer has also been marked.

Sample

The steel trap's jaws had caught the coyote midway across the foot. The pain must have been awful. Yet the coyote never stopped trying to tear loose. It had dug a circle about six inches (about 15.2 centimeters) deep, stretching the full length of the steel chain.

Two young boys out hiking saw this trapped coyote. They hurried to a nearby ranch. The ranch owner heard them out and came to help.

They held the coyote's neck down firmly with hoe handles. Then they opened the trap's jaws. The coyote slipped free. But the animal stayed there, just looking at its helpers. Perhaps it was wondering what makes some people demons and others saints.

The animal had to be gently nudged before it would leave. At last, it hobbled off a short distance. Then it turned, pausing to look again at the good people who had spared its life.

	Answer	Score
Mark the main idea	M	10
Mark the statement that is a detail	D	5
Mark the statement that is too narrow	N	5
Mark the statement that is too broad	B	5

a. Two young boys helped to free a trapped coyote.
[This statement is one that gathers all the important points. It gives a correct picture of the main idea in a brief way: (1) two young boys, (2) a trapped coyote, and (3) freeing it.]

b. Kind hearts set free a doomed coyote.
[This statement is too broad. It doesn't state *who* set the coyote free. It doesn't tell *why* it was doomed.]

c. Hoe handles were used to hold the coyote down.
[This is just one of many details found in the passage. It has little to do with the passage as a whole.]

d. A steel trap was opened to set a coyote free.
[Opening the trap is *part* of the main idea. But any main idea statement must give the chief actors credit. It must mention the two boys who set the coyote free.]

Getting the Most Out of This Book

The following steps could be called "tricks of the trade." Your teachers might call them "rules for learning." It doesn't matter what they are called. What does matter is that they work.

Think About the Title

A famous language expert told me a "trick" to use when I read. "The first thing to do is to read the title. Then spend a few moments thinking about it."

Writers spend much time thinking up good titles. They try to pack a lot of meaning into them. It makes sense, then, for you to spend a few seconds trying to dig out some meaning. These few moments of thought will give you a head start on a passage.

Thinking about the title can help you in another way, too. It helps you concentrate on a passage before you begin reading. Why does this happen? Thinking about the title fills your head full of thoughts about the passage. There's no room for anything else to get in to break concentration.

The Dot System

Here is a method that will speed up your reading. It also builds comprehension at the same time.

Spend a few moments with the title. Then read *quickly* through the passage. Next, without looking back, answer the six questions by placing a dot in the box next to each answer of your choice. The dots will be your "unofficial" answers. For the main idea question (question six), place your dot in the box next to the statement that you think is the main idea.

The dot system helps by making you think hard on your first, *fast* reading. The practice you gain by trying to grasp and remember ideas makes you a stronger reader.

The Check-Mark System

You have now answered all of the questions with a dot. Next, read the passage once more *carefully*. This time, make your final answer to each question with a check mark (✓). Go to each question. Then, place a check mark in the box next to the answer of your choice. The answers with the check marks are the ones that will count toward your score.

Now answer the main idea question. Follow the steps that are on the question page. Use a capital letter to mark your final answer to each part of the main idea question.

The Diagnostic Chart

Now move your final answers to the Diagnostic Chart on page 102. Use the column of boxes under number *1* for the answers to the first passage. Use the column of boxes under number *2* for the answers to the second passage, and so on.

Write the letter of your answer in the *upper* part of each block.

Correct your answers using the Answer Key on pages 100 and 101. When scoring your answers, do *not* use an *x* for *incorrect* or a *c* for *correct*. Instead, use this method. If your choice is correct, make no mark in the lower part of the answer block. If your choice is *in*correct, write the letter of the correct answer in the *lower* part of the block.

Thus, the answer column for each passage will show your incorrect answers. And it will also show the correct answers.

Your Total Comprehension Score

Go back to the passage you have just read. If you answered a question incorrectly, draw a line under the correct choice on the question page. Then write your score for each question in the circle provided. Add the scores to get your Total Comprehension Score.

Graphing Your Progress

After you have found your Total Comprehension Score, turn to the Progress Graph on page 103. Write your score in the box under the number for each passage. Then put an *x* along the line above the box to show your Total Comprehension Score. Join the *x*'s as you go. This will plot a line showing your progress.

Taking Corrective Action

Your incorrect answers give you a way to teach yourself how to read better. Take the time to study your wrong answers.

Go back to the question page. Read the correct answer (the one you have underlined) several times. With the correct answer in mind, go back to the passage itself. Read to see why the approved answer is better. Try to see where you made your mistake. Try to figure out why you chose a wrong answer.

Getting the Most Out of This Book

The Steps in a Nutshell

Here's a quick review of the steps to follow. Following these steps is the way to get the most out of each *Essential Skills* book. Be sure you have read and understood all of the "To the Student" section on pages 11 through 22 before you start.

1. **Think About the Title of the Passage.** Try to get all the meaning the writer put into it.
2. **Read the Passage Quickly.**
3. **Answer the Questions, Using the Dot System.** Use dots to mark your unofficial answers. Don't look back at the passage.
4. **Read the Passage Again — Carefully.**
5. **Mark Your Final Answers.** Put a check mark (✓) in the box to note your final answer. Use capital letters for each part of the main idea question.
6. **Mark Your Answers on the Diagnostic Chart.** Record your final answers in the upper blocks of the chart on page 102.
7. **Correct Your Answers.** Use the Answer Key on pages 100 and 101. If an answer is not correct, (a) write the correct answer in the lower block, beneath your wrong answer. Then (b) go back to the question page. Place a line under the correct answer.
8. **Find Your Total Comprehension Score.** Find this by adding up the points you earned for each question.
9. **Graph Your Progress.** Mark and plot your scores on the graph on page 103.
10. **Take Corrective Action.** Read your wrong answers. Read the passage once more. Try to figure out why you were wrong.

Passages and Questions

Titles of Passages

1. Do Animals Talk? 24
2. Eskimos 27
3. Light Enough To Fly 30
4. Fossils for the Future 33
5. The Test of Loyalty 36
6. Energy From the Sun 39
7. Jet Power 42
8. Driver Ants 45
9. How Sea Otters Stay Warm 48
10. Airborn Seeds 51
11. Friendly Snakes 54
12. Food for Survival 57
13. It's Raining Mule Deer! 60
14. The Turkey Family 63
15. Bobcats on the Prowl 66
16. Home Is What the Nest Is 69
17. The Great Salt Lake 72
18. The Food Chain 75
19. The Aphid Lion 78
20. The Hunter and the Hunted 81
21. The Rattlesnake 84
22. The Hungry Sea Anemone 87
23. Jaguar 90
24. Quilting Get-Togethers 93
25. When Winter Comes 96

1. Do Animals Talk?

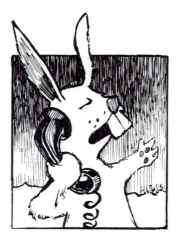 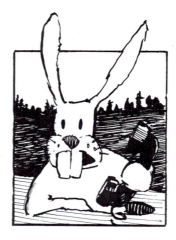

Many animals do talk to each other. But they do not use words. They use sound, odor, color and movement to communicate with one another.

Animals can tell each other if danger is coming. If you were to take a walk in the Rocky Mountains, you would be almost sure to hear a sharp, piercing whistle. It belongs to the yellow-bellied marmot.

When a marmot first sees an enemy coming, it warns its neighbors with a whistle. All the marmots stop what they are doing. They dive for their burrows among the rocks. When the danger has passed, one of the marmots will give the all-clear call — a low whistle. Its neighbors understand the message. Marmot life goes back to normal. Human words could not give messages as quickly or as plainly.

The little pika of the Rockies is a small, short-eared relative of the rabbit. It uses its voice to warn other pikas of danger. It is a skilled ventriloquist. Its whistle seems to come from a different place each time the pika calls. One time it sounds like it is far away. Then it seems to come from a pile of rocks or from inside a crevice. The bouncing sound fools enemies. It is said pikas can drive a hungry eagle crazy looking for them.

On the prairies, the black-tailed prairie dog has a warning bark. It tells others of the colony to look out for danger.

Animals give warnings in other ways, too. Pronghorn antelope have signal flags on their rumps. These are white patches of hair in the shape of a circle. The hair is short in the center and long as it spreads outward. When an antelope sights trouble, it quickly lifts its rump hairs so that the hairs catch the light and make flashes. The flashes are so bright that other antelope up to four miles (about 6.4 kilometers) away can see them. They flash warnings to others in turn.

?

| | Possible Score | Your Score |

1. What would be another good title for this passage?

   ☐ a. Warning Signals of Animals
   ☐ b. Mating Calls of the Wild
   ☐ c. How Animals Produce Sound
   ☐ d. Animals Can't Talk!

   Possible Score: 15

2. A skilled ventriloquist of the rockies is the

   ☐ a. marmot.
   ☐ b. pika.
   ☐ c. prairie dog.
   ☐ d. pronghorn.

   Possible Score: 15

3. It seems that many animals

   ☐ a. are quite talkative during mating.
   ☐ b. signal each other in time of danger.
   ☐ c. like to upset nearby neighbors.
   ☐ d. make ear-piercing whistles.

   Possible Score: 15

4. A "bouncing sound" is

   ☐ a. a whisper.
   ☐ b. a scream.
   ☐ c. an echo.
   ☐ d. an explosion.

   Possible Score: 15

5. A <u>piercing</u> whistle is very

   ☐ a. low pitched.
   ☐ b. soft.
   ☐ c. high pitched.
   ☐ d. dull.

   Possible Score: 15

6. Main Idea

	Answer	Score
Mark the main idea	M	10
Mark the statement that is a detail	D	5
Mark the statement that is too narrow	N	5
Mark the statement that is too broad	B	5

a. A pika is a small, short-eared relative of the rabbit which lives in the Rockies.

b. Many animals communicate with each other by using sounds, colors and movement to warn of danger.

c. The black-tailed prairie dog has a warning bark to tell others to look out for danger.

d. In their own individual ways, animals can understand one another.

Total Comprehension Score
(Add your scores and enter the total on the graph on page 103.)

Categories of Comprehension Questions

No. 1: Subject Matter	No. 4: Clarifying Devices
No. 2: Supporting Details	No. 5: Vocabulary in Context
No. 3: Conclusion	No. 6: Main Idea

2. Eskimos

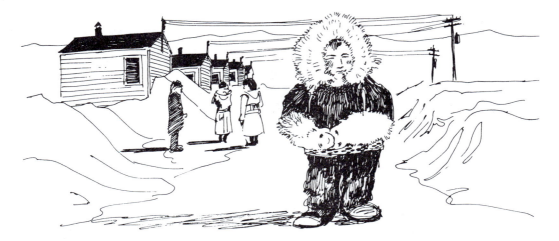

Eskimos have been called a warm, trusting and smart people. Some Eskimos live close to the land. Their village homes are not ice igloos but small wood or sod houses. No trees grow along the coast, so the Eskimos use coal for their fuel which they mine themselves. They also use branches from scrub willows and driftwood for fuel. For those who have the money to buy them, there are kerosene and fuel oil. Ice and snow are melted for the water supply. Some villages have electricity to make life more modern.

But Eskimos in the villages don't have the comfort of a well-stocked supermarket when they need food. The shopping list is made out just once a year. In July a ship brings what they have ordered.

Today, as in the past, many Eskimos depend on hunting and fishing to add to these supplies. But they no longer use dogsled teams to go from place to place. The snowmobile has now become a part of village life. It carries the hunters to track moose, caribou and rabbit.

Eskimo hunters have always made good use of the animals they kill. The meat is their food. The fur skins are used for their *parkas* (coats), *mukluks* (boots), rugs and sleeping bags. The tough skin of the intestines is made into rainwear. The *sinew* (tendons that hold bones together) is used for thread. The ivory is carved into needles and tools. For the tourist trade they also make items out of ivory, such as figures of seals, bears and birds.

In the summer when the sun is still shining at midnight, there are almost twenty-four hours of daylight. Families then move to fishing sites where they live in tents. Salmon fishing and berry picking are a big part of each day.

But the close-to-the-land life of the fishing sites and villages is disappearing. The white people's modern ideas are replacing the old ways. There is a sadness here for Eskimos trapped between the white people's way of life and a yearning to return to the quiet village they once knew.

?

	Possible Score	Your Score

1. This passage is about village Eskimo

   ☐ a. religion.
   ☐ b. ancestors.
   ☐ c. art.
   ☐ d. life.

   (15)

2. In summertime village Eskimos move

   ☐ a. further north.
   ☐ b. closer to fishing sites.
   ☐ c. to the mountains.
   ☐ d. to nearby islands.

   (15)

3. The writer suggests that the village Eskimo is being affected by

   ☐ a. a change in global climate.
   ☐ b. radioactive fallout.
   ☐ c. the Alaskan pipeline.
   ☐ d. the progress of white people.

   (15)

4. The first sentence tells one view of

   ☐ a. the Eskimo's nature.
   ☐ b. what the Eskimo looks like.
   ☐ c. the Eskimo's history.
   ☐ d. the home of the Eskimo.

   (15)

5. <u>Warm</u> people are

   ☐ a. smart.
   ☐ b. friendly.
   ☐ c. angry.
   ☐ d. trustworthy.

   (15)

6. Main Idea

	Answer	Score
Mark the main idea	M	10
Mark the statement that is a detail	D	5
Mark the statement that is too narrow	N	5
Mark the statement that is too broad	B	5

a. Village Eskimos carve ivory into needles, tools, and figures of animals.

b. Some groups of people do not live in modern ways.

c. Village Eskimos still live close to the land although their lifestyle is disappearing.

d. Fishing and hunting add to the village Eskimo's food supply.

Total Comprehension Score
(Add your scores and enter the total on the graph on page 103.)

Categories of Comprehension Questions

No. 1: Subject Matter	No. 4: Clarifying Devices
No. 2: Supporting Details	No. 5: Vocabulary in Context
No. 3: Conclusion	No. 6: Main Idea

3. Light Enough To Fly

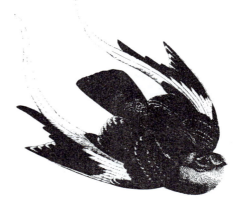

When you think of the fascinating things birds do, it is not surprising that humans have studied them for thousands of years. Even prehistoric people wrote picture stories about birds on the walls of caves.

How birds fly and stay up in the air has puzzled many people. Birds are amazingly light for their size. Little birds such as wrens and chickadees weigh less than twelve sheets of paper. Large hawks and owls seldom weigh more than six pounds (about 2.7 kilograms). What makes them so light?

A bird's streamlined covering weighs very little. We've all heard the expression "as light as a feather." Air trapped in the 2,000 feathers on a downy woodpecker's body not only decreases its weight compared to its size, but it also insulates against cold winter air. That is why birds fluff out their feathers on cold days.

A bird's bones are thin and not filled with marrow like ours. They are hollow! Air sacs reach from the lungs to different parts of the body and even into some of the bones. So, much of what is inside a bird is just air!

Look at the shape of the wings on a chicken, pheasant or chickadee. You will see that they are short and round. They are good for sudden, short bursts of speed. Swallow or killdeer wings are long and narrow — ideal for long, graceful flight.

As a bird flies, it moves its wings up and down with a peculiar motion that has a propeller effect. To stop, it reverses the motion. Humans discovered this method of stopping airplanes only recently, but birds have used it for millions of years.

?

1. What would be another good title for this passage?

   ☐ a. Different Shapes of Wings
   ☐ b. How a Bird Moves Its Wings
   ☐ c. As Light as a Feather
   ☐ d. Kinds of Bird Feathers

2. Some of the bones in a bird are filled with

   ☐ a. blood vessels.
   ☐ b. marrow.
   ☐ c. fat.
   ☐ d. air sacs.

3. The shape of a bird's wing

   ☐ a. does not help in flying.
   ☐ b. determines the kind of flight.
   ☐ c. helps in building nests.
   ☐ d. is like the elbow of a person.

4. The writer finds birds

   ☐ a. useless.
   ☐ b. fascinating.
   ☐ c. rather timid.
   ☐ d. intelligent.

5. <u>Graceful</u> flight is

   ☐ a. dangerous.
   ☐ b. clumsy.
   ☐ c. beautiful.
   ☐ d. careless.

6. Main Idea

	Answer	Score
Mark the main idea	M	10
Mark the statement that is a detail	D	5
Mark the statement that is too narrow	N	5
Mark the statement that is too broad	B	5

a. Birds fly and stay up in the air because they are light.

b. Birds are light and fly because air is trapped in their feathers.

c. Short, round wings are good for sudden, short bursts of speed.

d. Birds are able to fly and stay up in the air.

Total Comprehension Score
(Add your scores and enter the
total on the graph on page 103.)

Categories of Comprehension Questions

No. 1: Subject Matter	No. 4: Clarifying Devices
No. 2: Supporting Details	No. 5: Vocabulary in Context
No. 3: Conclusion	No. 6: Main Idea

4. Fossils for the Future

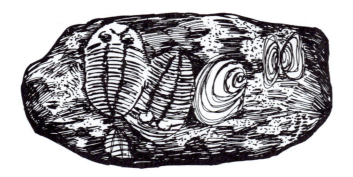

Think of an animal with a shell on the bottom of a shallow sea a long time ago — perhaps as long as 300 or 400 million years ago. It has no name, for there is no one to give it a name. No humans have yet appeared on the earth. Gulls do not yet fly over the water. There is only sea life — snails and clams, starfish, corals and soft-bodied creatures like jellyfish. Above the waves, the only sounds are the wind and the thunder. Below the waves, there is only silence.

Our sea-bottom creature lives its life. Then it dies as all living things must. Its soft body, if not eaten by scavengers, decays. In time all that is left is an empty shell lying in the mud and sand.

On the land nearby, air, rain and running water slowly wear away the surface. Rivers, muddy with millions of bits of rock, make their way to the sea. After some time, the shell is filled and covered with this sediment.

Many thousands of years pass. The mud and sand pack tightly around the shell as more sediment settles in the sea. Layer by layer the sediment piles up, but now something new is happening. Slowly the sea bottom is lifted. As it is lifted, the shallow sea that covers it drains back into the ocean.

A hundred million years pass, then one more hundred million. The mud and sand that were once a part of the sea bottom are now a part of the land. They are many hundred feet (hundreds of meters) above the sea. The layers of sediment that covered our shell have become solid rock. The shell is now a fossil buried deep within stone.

Air, rain and ice eat away at the rocks. Streams cut gullies. The decayed and crumbled rock is washed downhill. Much of it becomes silt and sand which are carried to the sea where they may bury more shells. As the rock is <u>eroded</u>, the surface of the ground gets lower and closer to our fossil. Two hundred million years of erosion at last reduce the rock to pieces. One of these pieces has the fossil shell in it. You may be lucky enough to find it in a stream bed or lake shore. When you do, you may be the first person in all of history to see it!

_____ **?** _____

	Possible Score	Your Score

1. This passage tells about fossils and how they are

   ☐ a. named.
   ☐ b. found.
   ☐ c. destroyed.
   ☐ d. formed.

   (15)   ◯

2. What is sediment?

   ☐ a. Streams
   ☐ b. Mud and sand
   ☐ c. Gullies
   ☐ d. The shoreline of a lake

   (15)   ◯

3. The writer suggests that

   ☐ a. humans have helped form fossils.
   ☐ b. fossils are hidden forever.
   ☐ c. there were no humans when fossils began forming.
   ☐ d. the pressure of the waves helps to destroy fossils.

   (15)   ◯

4. In the first sentence the writer is trying

   ☐ a. to make the reader part of the passage.
   ☐ b. to show how things decay.
   ☐ c. to be funny.
   ☐ d. to state an opinion.

   (15)   ◯

5. When a rock is <u>eroded</u>, it is

   ☐ a. turned into lava.
   ☐ b. finding its way to the sea.
   ☐ c. being worn down.
   ☐ d. becoming a fossil.

   (15)   ◯

6. Main Idea

	Answer	Score
Mark the main idea	M	10
Mark the statement that is a detail	D	5
Mark the statement that is too narrow	N	5
Mark the statement that is too broad	B	5

a. Layer after layer of mud and sand pack tightly around a shell to begin making it a fossil.

b. It takes many years to make a fossil.

c. It takes up to 300 to 400 million years of rock building and decaying to make a fossil.

d. Rivers bring bits of rock to the ocean.

Total Comprehension Score
(Add your scores and enter the total on the graph on page 103.)

Categories of Comprehension Questions

No. 1: Subject Matter	No. 4: Clarifying Devices
No. 2: Supporting Details	No. 5: Vocabulary in Context
No. 3: Conclusion	No. 6: Main Idea

5. The Test of Loyalty

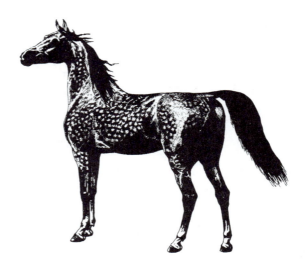

The stories of the Bedouin Arabs are filled with tales of horses that were loyal to their masters until death.

How did this fame for loyalty come about? Some who know the high intelligence of the Arabian horse will say that all it takes is training. It is true that this breed of horse is intelligent. You can see it in the horse's broad forehead. The horse has all the other marks, too. It has large eyes, so large that they bulge. They are set far to the side of the head, giving the horse wide vision. It is as if Nature had meant it to be able to see and know more than the average horse. And due to its intelligence, the Arabian horse learns quickly. It can be trained two to three times as fast as most other breeds.

Those who really know the Arabian horse, and its Bedouin masters, will be quick to say: "Yes, you can train the Arabian horse to do tricks. But you can't train loyalty into any horse. Loyalty must be bred into a horse. And it takes years and years to do that."

The speaker had in mind a custom of the Arabs. A herd of horses is placed inside a fenced field in view of water. There the horses are kept without food or water, day after day, until they are almost crazed. At last the horses cannot stand it any longer. Then the gates are thrown wide open. The horses make a mad dash for the river. At the very instant that they reach the water's edge and before a drop has been gulped, a horn is sharply blown for assembly. Only those horses that wheel right around and dash to the horn are kept for breeding. It is in this way that the Bedouin has built into the Arabian horse the priceless quality of loyalty.

?

	Possible Score	Your Score

1. The passage deals mainly with

   ☐ a. Arabs.
   ☐ b. training Arabian horses to jump.
   ☐ c. loyal Arabian horses.
   ☐ d. Arabian race horses.

   Possible Score: 15

2. The Arabian horse is

   ☐ a. weak.
   ☐ b. average.
   ☐ c. a slow learner.
   ☐ d. highly intelligent.

   Possible Score: 15

3. The last paragraph suggests that

   ☐ a. most of the horses die.
   ☐ b. this way of selection is still used.
   ☐ c. all the horses are kept.
   ☐ d. the horses are fed daily.

   Possible Score: 15

4. The custom of the Arabs that the passage describes

   ☐ a. is used to find water.
   ☐ b. has been used for about ten years.
   ☐ c. is used to select horses for breeding.
   ☐ d. is used to train intelligent horses.

   Possible Score: 15

5. The word <u>crazed</u> is closest in meaning to

   ☐ a. weak.
   ☐ b. sick.
   ☐ c. dead.
   ☐ d. crazy.

   Possible Score: 15

6. Main Idea

	Answer	Score
Mark the main idea	M	10
Mark the statement that is a detail	D	5
Mark the statement that is too narrow	N	5
Mark the statement that is too broad	B	5

a. The Arabs have bred loyalty into the Arabian horse.

b. The Arabian horse has a broad forehead.

c. Some animals can be bred for certain qualities.

d. The Arabs breed only the horses which pass the loyalty test.

Total Comprehension Score
(Add your scores and enter the total on the graph on page 103.)

Categories of Comprehension Questions

No. 1: Subject Matter	No. 4: Clarifying Devices
No. 2: Supporting Details	No. 5: Vocabulary in Context
No. 3: Conclusion	No. 6: Main Idea

6. Energy From the Sun

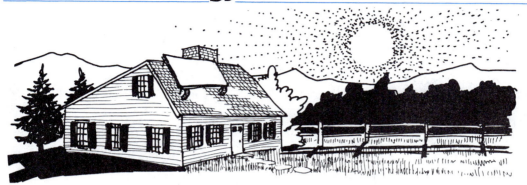

Sometimes you can't touch the car door handle or sit on the seat because they're so hot. This is solar energy. People can use this heat from the sun to keep warm and to get electricity.

We know that we will someday run out of fossil fuels. These are oil, gas and coal. So people are now spending lots of money to learn how to put nuclear energy to work for us. But we know that the radioactive wastes that come from using this kind of energy can be harmful.

We need a type of energy that will not pollute our air or water. It should not cost too much or run out. One of the sources people might use is the sun. Enough sunshine falls on the United States in one minute to give the whole country all the energy it needs for one day.

People want to collect some of this sun, or solar energy. Then we'll be able to make as much electricity as we need. And this won't make smog in our air or poison our water.

People could collect the sun's heat on big sun farms. A good place for a sun farm is in a desert. Here the sky is clear and there is plenty of sunshine and only a little rain. We could set up acres (hectares) of glass mirrors. The mirrors would focus the sun's rays on a special surface that would become very hot. Or we could put out many acres (hectares) of glass-covered collectors called *solar energy traps*. These transfer the sun's heat. The heat would melt a special metal. This melted metal would flow to a large tank of melted salt. The melted salt would then take the heat from the metal and hold it.

This stored heat could then be used like the heat we get from burning fossil fuels. It would make steam and turn motors to make electricity. There would even be enough heat to make steam in the night and on cloudy days.

The trouble is, collecting the sun's heat in these ways is costly right now. We need to find out how to make these methods cost less. Then people can have big sun farms in the deserts.

Two people in Colorado are making a solar energy collector. They hope it will be cheap enough for anyone to put on a house — either on the roof or in a wall. The inventors are making these solar collectors in kits for people who want to build their own.

?

	Possible Score	Your Score

1. What is the subject of this passage?

    ☐ a. Kinetic energy
    ☐ b. Nuclear energy
    ☐ c. Mechanical energy
    ☐ d. Solar energy

    15

2. The best place for a sun farm is the

    ☐ a. desert.
    ☐ b. seashore.
    ☐ c. mountains.
    ☐ d. forest.

    15

3. Scientists

    ☐ a. have finally found a safe way to use nuclear energy.
    ☐ b. know that fossil fuels will last forever.
    ☐ c. are still experimenting with energy from the sun.
    ☐ d. have found a cheap way to collect the sun's heat.

    15

4. The writer feels that nuclear energy

    ☐ a. will soon run out.
    ☐ b. is cheap.
    ☐ c. is clean.
    ☐ d. can be harmful.

    15

5. Smog is

    ☐ a. water vapor.
    ☐ b. polluted air.
    ☐ c. poisoned water.
    ☐ d. melted salt.

    15

6. Main Idea

	Answer	Score
Mark the main idea	M	10
Mark the statement that is a detail	D	5
Mark the statement that is too narrow	N	5
Mark the statement that is too broad	B	5

a. The sun's energy does not make smog.

b. We are looking for ways to collect the sun's energy to give us heat and electricity.

c. The sun is a good source of energy.

d. One way in which the sun's heat could be collected is on big sun farms in the desert.

Total Comprehension Score
(Add your scores and enter the total on the graph on page 103.)

Categories of Comprehension Questions

No. 1: Subject Matter	No. 4: Clarifying Devices
No. 2: Supporting Details	No. 5: Vocabulary in Context
No. 3: Conclusion	No. 6: Main Idea

7. Jet Power

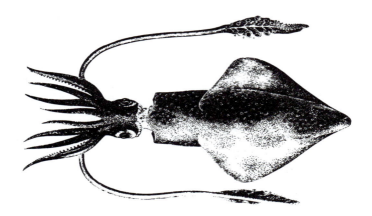

Some squid can swim so fast that they can leave water and glide through the air. The men on the famed ocean-crossing raft *Kon-Tiki* saw squid glide for fifty or sixty yards (about 45.8 to 55.9 meters). Squid have landed on ship decks twelve or more feet (about 3.7 meters or more) above the ocean surface. They make these leaps by firing a strong blast of water out through a nozzle on their body. Muscles can bend the nozzle to point in all directions. The jet of water sends the squid darting away like a jet plane hurtling into the sky. Then the squid can use its fins in a swift, brief glide.

Many squid have an ink sac. When they are attacked, they squirt a cloud of dark brown liquid into the water. This scares their enemies. It gives them a chance to escape. The cloud might have the shape of a real squid. Then it is called an *ink-dummy*.

Little is known about the eggs and babies of the giant squid. Many years ago some children were playing on an ocean beach in Jamaica. They ran to their father shouting, "We have found a great big sausage!" Their father happened to be a *zoologist,* an expert on animals. He saw that the object was five or six feet (about 1.5 to 1.8 meters) long and as big around as a bucket. He said that it could only be the egg case of a giant squid.

Some waterproof cameras hang in the sea on strong wires miles (kilometers) long. These might photograph a giant squid deep in the ocean. Or people cruising in a submarine in the blackness of the deep will suddenly see one in their headlights. Until then, people must depend on the sperm whale to tell them about the giant squid. Whales carry in their stomachs pieces of the giants from their homes a half-mile (about .8 kilometers) or more below the surface of the sea.

?

	Possible Score	Your Score

1. This passage tells us about

    ☐ a. mollusks.
    ☐ b. squid.
    ☐ c. minnows.
    ☐ d. sea worms.

    15

2. The famous raft that crossed the ocean was called

    ☐ a. Albatross.
    ☐ b. Arctic Tern.
    ☐ c. Kon-Tiki.
    ☐ d. Sandpiper.

    15

3. We can see that people have

    ☐ a. photographed every sea creature alive.
    ☐ b. invented a waterproof camera.
    ☐ c. many enemies below the surface of the ocean.
    ☐ d. never seen the giant squid.

    15

4. An ink sac is used for

    ☐ a. protection.
    ☐ b. mating.
    ☐ c. building a nest.
    ☐ d. hunting food.

    15

5. In this passage, the word firing means

    ☐ a. burning.
    ☐ b. containing.
    ☐ c. swallowing.
    ☐ d. shooting.

    15

6. Main Idea

	Answer	Score
Mark the main idea	M	10
Mark the statement that is a detail	D	5
Mark the statement that is too narrow	N	5
Mark the statement that is too broad	B	5

a. The squid is an ocean animal with many interesting habits.

b. The ocean contains many interesting creatures.

c. Squid travel by squeezing water out through their nozzle.

d. Underwater cameras may give us a photograph of a giant squid.

Total Comprehension Score
(Add your scores and enter the total on the graph on page 103.)

Categories of Comprehension Questions

No. 1: Subject Matter	No. 4: Clarifying Devices
No. 2: Supporting Details	No. 5: Vocabulary in Context
No. 3: Conclusion	No. 6: Main Idea

8. Driver Ants

The most ferocious of the army ants are the driver ants of Africa. There are tales about these ants eating huge pythons that could not flee because they were too stuffed with food. Another story tells of a lame elephant being eaten by ants. The drivers climbed into its trunk, ears and eyes. They covered it like a living blanket of jaws. In three days, only bones were left.

Ant birds follow the driver ants on their marches to catch the insects which the ants scare into flight. When the jungle natives hear the birds screeching, they quickly leave their villages. When they return, they find their homes empty of cockroaches, fleas and lice. The ants are nature's best bug killers. In one raid the ants can destroy as many as 100,000 insects.

The worker ants leave the nest to eat each day. As dusk comes, they return to their nest, and the whole colony begins marching to a new nesting site. The smallest workers had stayed in the nest during the day. Now they carry the larvae under their bodies. When the ants find a safe spot, they set up another camp for the night. The ants swarm together, and by late at night the camp may be over a yard wide.

The next morning a new raid begins. The workers pour out of the nest. By noon they have walked as far from the nest as the length of a football field. Nothing can stop their march except fire and large streams and rivers. They can cross small streams by hooking their legs together to form a living raft or bridge.

The raiding and camping lasts about two weeks. Then the wiggling larvae that the smaller workers have been carrying become still and spin cocoons. This quiets down the whole ant colony, and the workers stop their daily raids. The ants set up one more camp. They form a cluster in a sheltered spot and stay in this camp for a rest period of three weeks.

Inside this cluster the queen ant makes a nest and starts laying eggs — up to 15,000 a day! The eggs hatch and new larvae begin forming. Then new workers come out of the cocoons that had formed at the start of the rest period.

The new workers are full of energy. They spread excitement through the colony. They quickly join the older workers and start making small raids close to the nest. In a day or two, the whole colony is off again. For two more weeks they will be on the move. They attack and tear to pieces all creatures in their path.

?

| | Possible Score | Your Score |

1. This passage is about

   ☐ a. red ants.
   ☐ b. driver ants of Africa.
   ☐ c. carpenter ants.
   ☐ d. white ants.

   (15)

2. The raiding ants are followed by

   ☐ a. anteaters.
   ☐ b. elephants.
   ☐ c. ant birds.
   ☐ d. pythons.

   (15)

3. Army ants

   ☐ a. feed on small, tender plants.
   ☐ b. never stop to rest.
   ☐ c. leave the colony after they are born.
   ☐ d. live and work together.

   (15)

4. The writer mentions the lame elephant to show

   ☐ a. how merciless these ants can be.
   ☐ b. that army ants are kind.
   ☐ c. where most army ants live.
   ☐ d. the gentle nature of army ants.

   (15)

5. As used in this passage, a good synonym for <u>swarm</u> is

   ☐ a. eat.
   ☐ b. crowd.
   ☐ c. raid.
   ☐ d. run.

   (15)

6. Main Idea

	Answer	Score
Mark the main idea	M	10
Mark the statement that is a detail	D	5
Mark the statement that is too narrow	N	5
Mark the statement that is too broad	B	5

a. Driver ants follow a cycle of insect raids and rests.

b. Driver ants can cross small streams by hooking their legs together.

c. There are some natural bug killers found in the jungle of Africa.

d. Driver ants can kill up to 100,000 insects in a single raid.

Total Comprehension Score
(Add your scores and enter the total on the graph on page 103.)

Categories of Comprehension Questions

No. 1: Subject Matter	No. 4: Clarifying Devices
No. 2: Supporting Details	No. 5: Vocabulary in Context
No. 3: Conclusion	No. 6: Main Idea

9. How Sea Otters Stay Warm

Could you count the hairs on your head? There are most likely 100,000 of them. That's about 2,000 hairs to every square inch (almost three square centimeters). If you counted a hair each second, it would take nearly twenty-eight hours to count them all. That's a lot of hair. But even that much hair is like being bald compared to the amount of hair the sea otter has.

A big male otter might have 600 million hairs on its body. That's about 650 thousand in just a square inch (less than three square centimeters)!

The sea otter needs every one of those hairs! It lives in the cold waters of the North Pacific. It doesn't have <u>blubber</u> as whales do to keep it warm. When it swims, its fur traps air so that the cold water does not get in to wet and chill its skin. This same fur coat is kept all year long. It isn't shed, or "molted."

Besides its fur coat, the sea otter depends on energy to keep warm. The fuel of the animal furnace is food. Each day, each otter must eat twenty to thirty percent of its body weight in rich protein food. That's the same as a seventy-five pound (about 34 kilogram) child eating a fifteen-pound (about 7.8 kilogram) steak!

This animal has several problems at sea. It isn't nearly as good a swimmer as a seal or whale, and it can dive only about 150 feet (about 45.7 meters) deep. That is why sea otters must stay near shore where they can easily reach the bottom to get their food.

This means it can live only in a small part of the ocean — near shore. Yet, even here, the otters are still in danger from humans.

Pollution and oil spills are perhaps their biggest threat today. Boat propellers sometimes cut them badly as they float in the water. Some abalone fishers fear the sea otters are "eating up" their business. They would like to reduce the number of otters. But with proper care and protection, these gentle weasels will remain in the seas for a long time to come.

?

	Possible Score	Your Score

1. This passage is mainly about

    ☐ a. the sea otter's fur.
    ☐ b. the eating habits of the sea otter.
    ☐ c. where sea otters live.
    ☐ d. the sea otter's young.

    (15)   ◯

2. The biggest threat to otters today is

    ☐ a. disease.
    ☐ b. cold weather.
    ☐ c. over hunting.
    ☐ d. pollution.

    (15)   ◯

3. Otters live in shallow water because

    ☐ a. there is too much seaweed in deep water.
    ☐ b. deep water has no light.
    ☐ c. they are not good at making deep dives.
    ☐ d. deep water is too cold.

    (15)   ◯

4. The "fuel of the animal furnace" is

    ☐ a. food.
    ☐ b. energy.
    ☐ c. warmth.
    ☐ d. water.

    (15)   ◯

5. Another word for blubber is

    ☐ a. fins.
    ☐ b. fat.
    ☐ c. scales.
    ☐ d. bone.

    (15)   ◯

6. Main Idea

	Answer	Score
Mark the main idea	M	10
Mark the statement that is a detail	D	5
Mark the statement that is too narrow	N	5
Mark the statement that is too broad	B	5

a. Nature has provided ways for the sea otter to keep warm.

b. Sea otters can dive only about 150 feet (about 45.7 meters).

c. A sea otter has 600 million hairs on its body to keep it warm.

d. The sea otter depends on its hairy coat and energy from food to keep warm.

Total Comprehension Score
(Add your scores and enter the total on the graph on page 103.)

Categories of Comprehension Questions

No. 1: Subject Matter	No. 4: Clarifying Devices
No. 2: Supporting Details	No. 5: Vocabulary in Context
No. 3: Conclusion	No. 6: Main Idea

10. Airborne Seeds

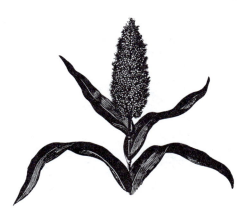

Seeds would not grow very well if they fell only under the parent plant. They would have to compete with the parent for water, light and minerals from the soil. It is much better for any species to be able to scatter its seeds far and wide. The seeds will then have a chance to find the best germinating conditions. Plants scatter their seeds in many ways.

A cottonwood tree has a tuft of silky fuzz for lifting its seeds on the wind. Seeds that have a tuft of fuzz fall to the ground very slowly. The slightest breeze has a chance to carry them far away before they strike the soil. Some airborne seeds can float many miles before landing.

Thistle, milkweed and cattail also have tufts of silk. Willows have tufts, too. But they have small and delicate seeds that soon die if they do not lodge in a place right for germination. Most other seeds carried by tufts of silk are stronger. They can stand many days of harsh conditions and still germinate.

Maples are perhaps the best known plants that have winged seeds. When the wind loosens the fruits of the maple with their seeds, they come spiraling to earth. Many land where they cannot grow — in the street, on the sidewalk, on roofs or in gutters. Others sift down between the sidewalk and the lawn, into the grass or under shrubs and germinate.

Catalpa seeds grow tightly packed in a long, slender pod. Every seed has a wing on each side. When the pod finally splits, these seeds may spin and tumble a long way before they settle to the ground.

A few trees bear their seeds in thin, papery pods that drift in the wind. The redbud is one. The wind rolls these seed pods for hundreds of feet (hundreds of meters) before they come to rest against a shrub or fence. There they nestle into the soil, germinate and, if conditions are right, begin to grow.

_____ **?** _____

	Possible Score	Your Score

1. What would be another good title for this passage?

   ☐ a. Seeds — Food for Thought
   ☐ b. Small Delicate Seeds
   ☐ c. Seeds and Sunlight
   ☐ d. The Scattering of Seeds   15   ◯

2. The best known plant that has winged seeds is the

   ☐ a. maple tree.
   ☐ b. milkweed.
   ☐ c. thistle.
   ☐ d. cottonwood tree.   15   ◯

3. In order to reproduce, the plants in this passage depend upon

   ☐ a. water.
   ☐ b. the wind.
   ☐ c. humans.
   ☐ d. seed explosions.   15   ◯

4. A "tuft of silky fuzz" would feel

   ☐ a. hard.
   ☐ b. soft.
   ☐ c. wet.
   ☐ d. bumpy.   15   ◯

5. A <u>delicate</u> seed is

   ☐ a. papery.
   ☐ b. tough.
   ☐ c. silky.
   ☐ d. frail.   15   ◯

6. Main Idea

	Answer	Score
Mark the main idea	M	10
Mark the statement that is a detail	D	5
Mark the statement that is too narrow	N	5
Mark the statement that is too broad	B	5

a. Some airborne seeds can float many feet (many meters) before they land.

b. The wind carries many seeds to places where they can grow.

c. New plants can grow far from their parent plants.

d. A cottonwood tree has a tuft of silk for floating its seeds on the wind.

Total Comprehension Score
(Add your scores and enter the total on the graph on page 103.)

Categories of Comprehension Questions

No. 1: Subject Matter	No. 4: Clarifying Devices
No. 2: Supporting Details	No. 5: Vocabulary in Context
No. 3: Conclusion	No. 6: Main Idea

11. Friendly Snakes

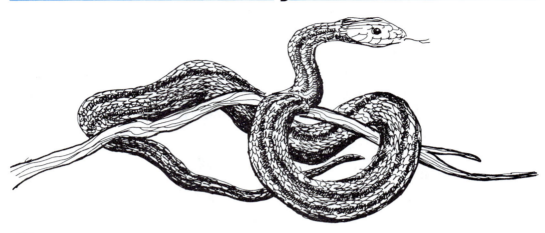

Garter snakes and other nonpoisonous snakes would never come up to you and shake hands. How could they even if they wanted to? But when you get to know them, they are so likeable you can call them your friends.

Have you ever turned over a rock and met a garter snake? There are more garters found in more places than any other snake in North America. They come in many colors and patterns, but you'll never mistake that friendliness!

Mole snakes are friendly, too. But when a hungry mole snake meets another snake, it may do a very unfriendly thing — *eat* the other snake! The mole snake eats even poisonous snakes. It is not harmed by their bite.

Mole snakes live all over the southeastern United States, but you may not find many. Why? Because, as you may guess from their name, they burrow in the ground. After a hard rain, they may come wiggling up like giant earthworms.

Yellow-bellied racers, which live in the United States Midwest, are hard to find, too, but for a different reason. They can zip out of sight so fast you'd never know they were near. These speedy rat-eaters have no trouble outrunning *you,* but hawks and owls find them easy prey.

To find a rough green snake you have to look up, not down. The rough green is an expert tree climber who lives in the southeastern states. It looks so much like a vine twisting among the leaves that it has the nickname "vine snake."

Do you have a shy friend? You do if you know the scarlet king snake. But why would a shy snake show off in such a fancy costume? It copies the colors of the deadly coral snake which is its southeastern neighbor. Enemies can't tell the difference, so they leave *both* snakes alone.

If you spend enough time looking, you may meet lots of gentle, harmless snakes where you live. Just remember — even though they don't (and can't) slither up and shake hands, they still are very good friends.

?

| | Possible Score | Your Score |

1. What is this passage about?

   ☐ a. Snake skins
   ☐ b. Nonpoisonous snakes
   ☐ c. Dangerous snakes
   ☐ d. Uses of snake venom

   (15)   ◯

2. Which of the following snakes can be found climbing a tree?

   ☐ a. The garter snake
   ☐ b. The mole snake
   ☐ c. The yellow-bellied racer
   ☐ d. The rough green snake

   (15)   ◯

3. A yellow-bellied racer feeds mostly on

   ☐ a. rats.
   ☐ b. birds.
   ☐ c. insects.
   ☐ d. frogs.

   (15)   ◯

4. The scarlet king snake looks like the deadly coral snake. This is how the scarlet king

   ☐ a. traps enemies.
   ☐ b. communicates.
   ☐ c. protects itself.
   ☐ d. decorates itself.

   (15)   ◯

5. An <u>expert</u> tree climber

   ☐ a. is very poor at tree climbing.
   ☐ b. dislikes trees.
   ☐ c. climbs only dead trees.
   ☐ d. is good at climbing trees.

   (15)   ◯

6. Main Idea

	Answer	Score
Mark the main idea	M	10
Mark the statement that is a detail	D	5
Mark the statement that is too narrow	N	5
Mark the statement that is too broad	B	5

a. Many creatures are harmless to humans.

b. Garter snakes are nonpoisonous.

c. There are many gentle, harmless, friendly snakes.

d. The scarlet king snake copies the colors of the coral snake.

Total Comprehension Score
(Add your scores and enter the total on the graph on page 103.)

Categories of Comprehension Questions

No. 1: Subject Matter	No. 4: Clarifying Devices
No. 2: Supporting Details	No. 5: Vocabulary in Context
No. 3: Conclusion	No. 6: Main Idea

12. Food for Survival

Water is necessary to survival. The other necessity in a survival situation is food. There are two kinds, plant and animal. Plant foods are hard to teach people about for there are thousands of poisonous plants in the world. Some are so deadly that one bite could be fatal. A good example is one you probably have had in your home — the poinsettia. One leaf could kill a child. Some parts of many plants are edible, while other parts are poisonous. For example, rhubarb stems are good but the leaves are deadly. The May apple is good to eat but the rest of the plant has sixteen poisons in it. Never eat a plant unless you are certain you know what it is. In military survival training, the recruits are taught about ten plants that are safe to eat. They are told to avoid the others. The best advice is to learn from local inhabitants.

Anyhow, don't worry — your chances of starving to death are very slim. You can eat anything in the animal kingdom except two things, and you're not likely to run across either of these. One is polar bear liver. It is poisonous because it contains so much vitamin A. One very small piece might be good for you, as a vitamin A pill is. However, if you ate a large piece, all of your hair would fall out. Sometimes Eskimo dogs eat too much, causing their hair to fall out, and they freeze to death. A large portion could make you extremely sick or even be fatal.

There are three fish that are poisonous when found around coral islands. In other oceans and other parts of the world, they are good to eat. However, around coral islands they feed on something that makes them deadly poisonous. Easy to remember by their names, they are the puffer fish, the parrot fish and the trigger fish. When out of the water, the puffer fish puffs up like a big balloon. The parrot fish has a head that looks like that bird. The trigger fish has two fins on its back. One is shaped like the hammer of a gun, and beneath it is a smaller fin like a trigger. If you pull the trigger fin, the hammer fin comes down with a snap or click, and that's how this fish gets its name.

_____ **?** _____

	Possible Score	Your Score

1. The subject of this passage is

   ☐ a. herbs and spices.
   ☐ b. nongreen plants.
   ☐ c. poisonous foods.
   ☐ d. foreign delicacies.

   15

2. A polar bear's liver contains

   ☐ a. iron.
   ☐ b. vitamin A.
   ☐ c. niacin.
   ☐ d. vitamin C.

   15

3. The last paragraph suggests that

   ☐ a. some fish are poisonous because of what they eat.
   ☐ b. poinsettia leaves are poisonous.
   ☐ c. the May apple is good to eat.
   ☐ d. vitamin A can cause hair to fall out.

   15

4. The parrot fish looks like a

   ☐ a. snake.
   ☐ b. butterfly.
   ☐ c. bird.
   ☐ d. dog.

   15

5. If something is <u>fatal</u>, it is

   ☐ a. good to eat.
   ☐ b. careless.
   ☐ c. lively.
   ☐ d. deadly.

   15

6. Main Idea

	Answer	Score
Mark the main idea	M	10
Mark the statement that is a detail	D	5
Mark the statement that is too narrow	N	5
Mark the statement that is too broad	B	5

a. A tiny piece of polar bear liver is as good for you as a vitamin A pill.

b. In a survival situation, many things found in nature can be harmful.

c. Polar bear liver is poisonous because it contains so much vitamin A.

d. Many plants are poisonous, but only polar bear liver and three coral island fish are poisonous animals.

Total Comprehension Score
(Add your scores and enter the total on the graph on page 103.)

Categories of Comprehension Questions

No. 1: Subject Matter	No. 4: Clarifying Devices
No. 2: Supporting Details	No. 5: Vocabulary in Context
No. 3: Conclusion	No. 6: Main Idea

13. It's Raining Mule Deer!

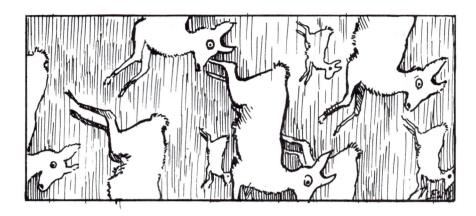

The spotted <u>fawns</u> of mule deer are adorable. One to three fawns are born to each doe in late May, June or July. They grow up quickly and may have their own babies when they are two or three years old.

This can lead to a fast rise in the number of mule deer. On one farm, for example, a man had three deer in an area that was fenced in. Six years later he had forty-four deer!

Before white people came to North America, Indians hunted the mule deer. They ate the meat. They made many useful things from the animals' hides, bones, antlers, teeth and sinews.

Then, in the late 1880s, white people began killing the mule deer for their hides. In British Columbia thousands were shipped out and sold for twenty-five cents each! So, in some parts of Canada, the mule deer became harder and harder to find. Out on the Great Plains it was almost wiped out. It has never come back in some provinces and states.

But in Arizona, just the opposite happened. A game reserve was started in the Kaibab National Forest near the Grand Canyon. In 1906 there were about 3,000 mule deer living in 1,000 square miles (about 1,610 kilometers). No hunting was allowed. Big enemies — such as panthers, wolves, coyotes and bears — were killed. In less than twenty years, it wasn't raining cats and dogs, it was raining mule deer! There were 30,000 of them!

The result was that the little fawns were sickly. In winter, hundreds of animals starved to death. Deer food was almost gone, and the soil and plants were crushed from so many deer hooves walking over them.

This taught game biologists and other people a good lesson. They saw that deer, like other kinds of animals, must live in balance with their food supply. Hunting was again allowed, and the deer herd was trimmed down. In time, both the deer and the plants became healthy again.

?

| | Possible Score | Your Score |

1. This passage is about the mule deer

   ☐ a. and its family life.
   ☐ b. as a meat-eating animal.
   ☐ c. population.
   ☐ d. and its expensive hide.

   Possible Score: 15

2. Mule deer have babies when they are

   ☐ a. 1 year old.
   ☐ b. 2 or 3 years old.
   ☐ c. 4 years old.
   ☐ d. 8 or 9 years old.

   Possible Score: 15

3. When a herd of animals becomes too large, many of its members

   ☐ a. become tame.
   ☐ b. begin fighting.
   ☐ c. leave the herd.
   ☐ d. starve to death.

   Possible Score: 15

4. In less than 20 years, it was raining mule deer. This means

   ☐ a. the deer found water.
   ☐ b. there were too many mule deer.
   ☐ c. many deer dislike water.
   ☐ d. mule deer live in swamps.

   Possible Score: 15

5. A <u>fawn</u> is

   ☐ a. a male deer.
   ☐ b. an old deer.
   ☐ c. a female deer.
   ☐ d. a young deer.

   Possible Score: 15

6. Main Idea

	Answer	Score
Mark the main idea	M	10
Mark the statement that is a detail	D	5
Mark the statement that is too narrow	N	5
Mark the statement that is too broad	B	5

a. Animal populations are not always in balance with their surroundings.

b. The mule deer population has been overhunted in some areas and overprotected in others.

c. Mule deer multiplied so fast in the Kaibab National forest that deer food was running out.

d. One to three mule deer fawns are born to each doe in late May, June or July.

Total Comprehension Score
(Add your scores and enter the total on the graph on page 103.)

Categories of Comprehension Questions

No. 1: Subject Matter	No. 4: Clarifying Devices
No. 2: Supporting Details	No. 5: Vocabulary in Context
No. 3: Conclusion	No. 6: Main Idea

14. The Turkey Family

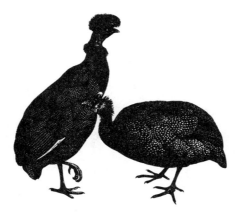

It had been twenty-eight days since the turkey hen had laid her last egg. Now early in the morning the first baby turkey, or *poult,* had hatched. By noon, five more had wriggled themselves free from their shells.

By midafternoon the rest of the clutch had hatched. A few hours later, nine poults followed their mother toward the creek for their first drink of water.

For the next few weeks the poults snuggled under their mother's wings for shelter. If they became chilled or wet, they would die. But it turned out that the long days of June were warm, and there was enough food. The poults grew quickly.

A hunting hawk flew low over the woodland, looking for the slightest movement. It came to a clearing where the turkey family was feeding on insects. The hawk was so swift that the hen didn't see it.

The hawk dropped down, swinging its legs forward, delivering a bone-cracking blow to the smallest poult. It sank its claws deep into the poult's back. The poult's cries shattered the silence. Then suddenly it became limp and quiet. Before the hen could help the poult, the hawk flew away with its food.

All summer long the turkey family fed on tender grass, insects, berries, snails and earthworms. By the time fall arrived, beechnuts and acorns became part of their diet. Now they were almost full-grown. Even so, the little flock would stay together until the spring and the start of the mating season.

_____ **?** _____

	Possible Score	Your Score

1. The members of the turkey family talked about most are the

   ☐ a. males.
   ☐ b. hens.
   ☐ c. babies.
   ☐ d. leaders.

   (15)　○

2. How long does it take for turkey eggs to hatch?

   ☐ a. A few days
   ☐ b. 1 week
   ☐ c. 28 days
   ☐ d. 2 months

   (15)　○

3. After reading this passage, we can guess that an enemy of the turkey is

   ☐ a. the hawk.
   ☐ b. the weasel.
   ☐ c. people.
   ☐ d. the eagle.

   (15)　○

4. What is happening in the first paragraph?

   ☐ a. The turkeys are fighting
   ☐ b. Baby turkeys are hatching
   ☐ c. The male turkey is eating
   ☐ d. A turkey has just been killed

   (15)　○

5. By midafternoon the rest of the clutch had hatched. As used here, a *clutch* is

   ☐ a. a flock of turkeys.
   ☐ b. a steel shift.
   ☐ c. a tight grip.
   ☐ d. a set of eggs to be hatched.

   (15)　○

6. Main Idea

	Answer	Score
Mark the main idea	M	10
Mark the statement that is a detail	D	5
Mark the statement that is too narrow	N	5
Mark the statement that is too broad	B	5

a. In the wild, a turkey hen may have as many as 9 poults.

b. Baby turkeys grow quickly, but many dangers threaten their family unit.

c. By the time fall arrives, the turkey poults are almost full-grown.

d. Many baby animals must survive the threats of enemies to grow up.

Total Comprehension Score
(Add your scores and enter the total on the graph on page 103.)

Categories of Comprehension Questions

No. 1: Subject Matter	No. 4: Clarifying Devices
No. 2: Supporting Details	No. 5: Vocabulary in Context
No. 3: Conclusion	No. 6: Main Idea

15. Bobcats on the Prowl

A six-inch (about 15-centimeter) tail gives the bobcat its name. Its short tail is unlike all other North American cats' except its larger northern cousin, the Canada lynx. Most bobcats weigh from fifteen to twenty-five pounds (about 6.8 to 11.3 kilograms). They stand just over a foot (about .30 meters) tall at the shoulder. A really large one may weigh close to forty pounds (about 18.1 kilograms).

A bobcat in search of food depends to a great extent on its keen eyesight. It can see in daylight as well as dark, though it does most of its hunting at night. Most of the cat's daylight hours are spent in hiding places.

The bobcat hunts the same area of land rather than covering great distances at one time. Each night it hunts a different small part of the large area with which it is familiar. It may walk and trot five or six miles (about 8.1 or 9.7 kilometers), wandering about and crossing its own trail. It never goes more than a mile (about 1.6 kilometers) from its starting point. This way of hunting insures the bobcat a constant food supply. It is not eliminating all the small animals on which it feeds at one time.

In the north, snow will make tracking the bobcat easy. A tracker can puzzle out its nightly route. It moves from one spot of dense cover to another, sniffing the trails of small animals. It seems rarely to track down one animal. Rather, it goes from trail to trail until its keen eye catches a movement close by. Sometimes it may pick a spot in which to lie in wait for passing prey. If it cannot catch an animal in a couple of eight-foot (about 2.4 meter) bounds, it gives up and looks for another.

Cottontails are the major part of the bobcat's diet. But the cats eat whatever food is most abundant and easiest to get. When the rabbit supply is low, bobcats hunt other small animals for food.

Young bobcats are born in early spring. The female will settle for just about any type of den in which to raise her young. A hollow tree or a rock crevice may be used, or any other place that is dry and well hidden. Most bobcats breed in late winter. The kittens are born about two months after mating. There may be as many as seven "kits". But the usual number is two or three. They are weaned when three months old. The one or two kittens which live stay with the mother until fall, learning from her the skills of survival.

?

	Possible Score	Your Score

1. What would be another good title for this passage?

   ☐ a. Facts about Bobcats
   ☐ b. The Canadian Lynx
   ☐ c. How To Catch a Cat
   ☐ d. Bounty for Bobcats   15   ◯

2. A really large bobcat may weigh close to

   ☐ a. 10 pounds (about 4.5 kilograms).
   ☐ b. 20 pounds (about 9.1 kilograms).
   ☐ c. 30 pounds (about 13.6 kilograms).
   ☐ d. 40 pounds (about 18.1 kilograms).   15   ◯

3. We can conclude from this passage that bobcats

   ☐ a. are becoming extinct in the snow-covered areas of the North.
   ☐ b. are able to see quite well at night.
   ☐ c. have a poor sense of direction.
   ☐ d. consume a great number of rabbits each day.   15   ◯

4. The bobcat gets its name from its

   ☐ a. mating call.
   ☐ b. appearance.
   ☐ c. dietary habits.
   ☐ d. nature.   15   ◯

5. Eliminating means

   ☐ a. increasing in number.
   ☐ b. tracking down.
   ☐ c. getting rid of.
   ☐ d. hiding from.   15   ◯

6. Main Idea

	Answer	Score
Mark the main idea	M	10
Mark the statement that is a detail	D	5
Mark the statement that is too narrow	N	5
Mark the statement that is too broad	B	5

a. A bobcat follows trails until its eye catches a movement.

b. Bobcats obtain their food by hunting.

c. As many as 7 kittens are born in a bobcat litter.

d. A bobcat has special habits for hunting.

Total Comprehension Score
(Add your scores and enter the total on the graph on page 103.)

Categories of Comprehension Questions

No. 1: Subject Matter	No. 4: Clarifying Devices
No. 2: Supporting Details	No. 5: Vocabulary in Context
No. 3: Conclusion	No. 6: Main Idea

16. Home Is What the Nest Is

To many of us, a bird nest is simply a cup of grass or twigs. But the naturalist knows that bird nests are as varied as the creatures that make them. A few birds build no nest at all. Murres, for instance, merely place their eggs on narrow ledges on seaside cliffs. Nighthawks lay theirs on bare, gravelly ground or on gravel roofs.

The shore-loving black skimmer digs a hollow in the sand and calls it a nest. Most plovers line their hollows with broken clam shells. Grebes, being almost helpless on land, lay their eggs on floating plants in the water.

Many birds place their eggs in natural holes. The rough-winged swallow shelters its eggs in cliff-side crannies. The turkey vulture chooses caves or hollow logs. The kingfisher tunnels two to five feet (about .61 to 1.5 meters) into a high stream bank. Flocks of bank swallows riddle sand banks with holes that lead to nests lined with feathers. They enter and exit with great speed.

Some birds are skillful potters. Cliff swallows form flask-shaped nests of mud pellets beneath the ledges of rocky cliffs or beneath the eaves of a barn. Barn swallows stick their feather-lined mud cups to barn timbers.

Long-billed marsh wrens weave small, globular nests of grass with an entrance hole in the side. Strangely, the males build dummy nests which are never used.

Unique among nests are those of the chimney swifts. Many years ago their brackets of twigs were attached to the inside of hollow trees. But chimneys are now preferred nesting sites. Twigs, snapped off in flight, are glued together with the bird's sticky saliva which hardens into a varnishlike substance.

The smallest nests are those of the hummingbirds. Most of them fashion a cup out of plant fuzz. They shingle it with lichens and bind it together with spider webs. The cavity is about one and one-fifth inches (about 30.6 millimeters) across. The eagle's aerie, on the other hand, is our largest nest. Its mass of huge sticks might be gathered for twenty or thirty years. One of the biggest known of these measured over eight feet (about 2.4 meters) across by twelve feet (about 3.7 meters) deep. It was guessed to weigh nearly two tons (about 1.8 tonnes). No matter what the nest looks like, it's still home to our feathered friends.

?

	Possible Score	Your Score

1. What would be another good title for this passage?

   ☐ a. How to Fool a Bird
   ☐ b. Hollow Tree Dwellers
   ☐ c. Why Birds Build Nests
   ☐ d. Different Kinds of Bird Nests

   (15)

2. Murres build their nests

   ☐ a. on narrow ledges.
   ☐ b. in gravel banks.
   ☐ c. in hollowed-out trees.
   ☐ d. on floating vegetation.

   (15)

3. We can conclude that grebes

   ☐ a. build their nests on gravel roofs.
   ☐ b. lay only a few eggs.
   ☐ c. live on or near water.
   ☐ d. build the smallest bird nest.

   (15)

4. A shore-loving bird lives

   ☐ a. in dry desert areas.
   ☐ b. on rocky ledges.
   ☐ c. in mountain areas.
   ☐ d. near the ocean.

   (15)

5. An <u>aerie</u> is an eagle's

   ☐ a. eggs.
   ☐ b. prey.
   ☐ c. nest.
   ☐ d. young.

   (15)

6. Main Idea

	Answer	Score
Mark the main idea	M	10
Mark the statement that is a detail	D	5
Mark the statement that is too narrow	N	5
Mark the statement that is too broad	B	5

a. Birds try to provide a home for their eggs.

b. Long-billed marsh wrens weave small, round nests with an entrance hole in the side.

c. Bank swallows enter and leave their nests with great speed.

d. Some birds lay their eggs in natural settings; others build nests in different ways.

Total Comprehension Score
(Add your scores and enter the total on the graph on page 103.)

Categories of Comprehension Questions

No. 1: Subject Matter	No. 4: Clarifying Devices
No. 2: Supporting Details	No. 5: Vocabulary in Context
No. 3: Conclusion	No. 6: Main Idea

17. The Great Salt Lake

Add five teaspoonfuls (about 25 milliliters) of salt to a glass of water. This will taste as salty as the sea. You would have to add at least five more teaspoonfuls (about 25 more milliliters) to get water as salty as that in Great Salt Lake.

All the rivers of the world are carrying salts and other minerals into the ocean. Water is always evaporating from the surface of the ocean. When the water leaves, the salts and other minerals are left behind. Through millions of years the seas have become salty. The same thing happened to what is now Great Salt Lake in Utah.

Great Salt Lake is fed by many rivers which carry salt into it. This is because they wash over the salt-bearing rocks of the region. But the Lake has no river flowing out of it. As some of its water evaporates, all the salts remain.

Each year one hundred tons (about 90 tonnes) of common table salt are taken from this long and placid lake.

Great Salt Lake has a special value for swimmers. They can float easily. As you may know, it is easier to float in the ocean than in fresh water. Great Salt Lake is even saltier than the ocean. So it is easier to float in.

There are no fish in the lake. Yet there are some twenty-four other forms of life. They are all small. They start with bacteria, algae and one-celled animals and move up to the three-eighths-inch-long (about 9.5 millimeters long) brine shrimp.

The birds attract many visitors. Seagulls are most common. They are part of early Mormon history. They saved the first settlers' crops from a plague of crickets.

The land to the east of Great Salt Lake is filled with birds through much of the year. One of the best-known big birds in the world — the pelican — can be found here. The great white pelican uses the Great Salt Lake for a home. It nests on Gunnison Island. This is one of the thirteen islands in the Great Salt Lake.

The adult pelicans fly a few miles (several kilometers) eastward to the freshwater marshes to get food. They swim side by side across the wide ponds and scoop up bills full of carp. Then, with a full load of fish, the pelicans fly back to Gunnison Island to feed birds which cannot yet fly.

?

	Possible Score	Your Score

1. This passage tells us

   ☐ a. about resort areas around the Great Salt Lake.
   ☐ b. why the Great Salt Lake is becoming smaller.
   ☐ c. when the Great Salt Lake was formed.
   ☐ d. many facts about the Great Salt Lake.

   15

2. How many islands are found in the Great Salt Lake?

   ☐ a. 10
   ☐ b. 13
   ☐ c. 20
   ☐ d. 23

   15

3. Pelicans fly a long distance from the Great Salt Lake to get food because

   ☐ a. the young must have a special diet.
   ☐ b. the Great Salt Lake is too small.
   ☐ c. pelicans eat ocean fish.
   ☐ d. there are no fish in the Great Salt Lake.

   15

4. The second paragraph tells us

   ☐ a. how the Great Salt Lake became salty.
   ☐ b. about the birdlife of the Great Salt Lake.
   ☐ c. how salt is taken from the Great Salt Lake.
   ☐ d. the size of the Great Salt Lake.

   15

5. When water <u>evaporates,</u> it changes from liquid into a

   ☐ a. solid.
   ☐ b. sand mixture.
   ☐ c. gas.
   ☐ d. mineral.

   15

6. Main Idea

	Answer	Score
Mark the main idea	M	10
Mark the statement that is a detail	D	5
Mark the statement that is too narrow	N	5
Mark the statement that is too broad	B	5

a. The Mormons were saved from a plague of crickets by seagulls.

b. Some bodies of water contain a great deal of salt.

c. Birds such as the pelican use the Great Salt Lake for a home, but feed elsewhere.

d. Great Salt Lake is much saltier than the ocean which affects the life forms in and around it.

Total Comprehension Score
(Add your scores and enter the total on the graph on page 103.)

Categories of Comprehension Questions

No. 1: Subject Matter	No. 4: Clarifying Devices
No. 2: Supporting Details	No. 5: Vocabulary in Context
No. 3: Conclusion	No. 6: Main Idea

18. The Food Chain

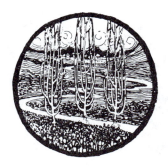

All life is tied in some way to energy from sunlight. Plants are the only livings things that can use this energy right from the sun. Their leaves are tiny factories. They use sunlight to make food from water and minerals in the soil and carbon dioxide in the air. This process is called *photosynthesis*.

Plants, in turn, feed all other living things. Animals can only use the sun's life-giving energy after plants have changed it into food. Animals that feed on plants are called *herbivores*. When these animals are eaten by other animals, the sun's energy is passed on again.

A butterfly sips nectar from a flower. This nectar contains the sun's energy in the form of sugars made by the plant. A dragonfly eats the butterfly. It, in turn, is eaten by a frog. The frog is caught by a watersnake. The snake is snatched up by a red-shouldered hawk. The hawk is called the final consumer because it is the last link in the chain. There is nothing which preys on it for food — while it is alive. But after it dies, tiny organisms break down its body into its basic chemicals. These chemicals are then taken up by plant roots and the food chain starts over again. So this chain of life is really a cycle, without a beginning or an ending.

People are members of many food chains. One of the simplest is plant-to-people. One example of this food chain takes place when people eat vegetables. When people eat meat or drink milk, they are part of a three-link chain: grass-to-cow-to-people.

The sad fact is that people disturb and sometimes even destroy the chains. We pollute rivers, lakes and the air that mean life to all. In doing so, we may damage food chains we know little or nothing about. But this we do know: each form of life, including humans, is linked to all others. Breaking links puts all life in danger.

?

	Possible Score	Your Score

1. The food chain passes on

    ☐ a. sickness.
    ☐ b. energy.
    ☐ c. light.
    ☐ d. water.   (15)   ◯

2. The process by which plants make food is called

    ☐ a. photosynthesis.
    ☐ b. herbivores.
    ☐ c. synthesis.
    ☐ d. chemicals.   (15)   ◯

3. Animals

    ☐ a. are not part of the food chain.
    ☐ b. are all meat-eaters.
    ☐ c. cannot change sunlight into food.
    ☐ d. damage the food chain by breaking the links. (15)   ◯

4. We can see that the food chain is

    ☐ a. poisonous.
    ☐ b. careless.
    ☐ c. useless.
    ☐ d. continuous.   (15)   ◯

5. <u>Organisms</u> are

    ☐ a. a kind of rock.
    ☐ b. rain, snow, sleet and hail.
    ☐ c. living things.
    ☐ d. chemicals.   (15)   ◯

6. Main Idea

	Answer	Score
Mark the main idea	M	10
Mark the statement that is a detail	D	5
Mark the statement that is too narrow	N	5
Mark the statement that is too broad	B	5

a. All life depends in one way or another on the sun.

b. Some animals get the sun's energy by eating plants.

c. The sun's energy is passed on to living things by the food chain.

d. Humans disturb and destroy food chains with pollution.

Total Comprehension Score
(Add your scores and enter the total on the graph on page 103.)

Categories of Comprehension Questions

No. 1: Subject Matter	No. 4: Clarifying Devices
No. 2: Supporting Details	No. 5: Vocabulary in Context
No. 3: Conclusion	No. 6: Main Idea

19. The Aphid Lion

One warm summer day a little, brown aphid lion pushed out of her eggshell. She climbed down the thin white <u>filament</u> to which her egg was attached and reached the midrib of a rose leaf. Right there she came face to face with a bright green aphid!

She had never seen an aphid before, but she instantly grabbed it in her hard pincer jaws and sucked out its life juices. It took less than one minute! She tossed aside the empty skin and grabbed another aphid. And then another. She ate ten aphids . . . twenty . . . fifty! A hundred! (As a matter of fact her giant appetite is the reason she is commonly called a "lion.") For two days she kept eating. Her skin grew tight so she stopped eating. Suddenly her skin started splitting behind her head. She drew back her head and pushed it through the slit. She tugged and pulled until her fat body and six thin legs were out of the tight covering.

Then she raced to another colony of soft, green aphids, and she ate them all, one by one. If she found no aphids, she sucked the juice from mealy bugs, thrips or mites. Sometimes she piled the remains of her victims on her back so that she looked like a walking trash pile. The aphid lion's big appetite helps keep garden insects in balance. This tiny insect is just one of nature's pesticides.

About two days later, when her second skin grew tight, she shed it, too. She gobbled another hundred or so aphids and slipped out of her third skin. The gobbling continued until she had shed a fourth and final skin.

After about ten days of eating bright green aphids and shedding skins, the little aphid lion crawled off to rest on the underside of a rose leaf. She spun a greenish white cocoon around herself and soon was completely within it.

Two summer weeks went by. One day she awoke all cramped inside the cocoon. She cut a round door in the silken roof above her head, pushed it open and pulled herself out into the bright summer world. Slowly and stiffly she crawled about. She began to move her new wings. They were thin, gauzy, pale-green, rainbow-tinted wings. During her sleep the greedy little aphid lion had become a delicate green, golden-eyed lacewing about half an inch (about 1.3 centimeters) long.

When darkness came she climbed a tall stalk of timothy grass. Her perfume drifted on the evening air. It had an unpleasant odor to all insects except male lacewings. One came at once to meet her. Soon after they had mated, the new green lacewing began to lay her eggs — one by one.

_____ **?** _____

		Possible Score	Your Score

1. This passage is about the growth of a

   ☐ a. moth.
   ☐ b. praying mantis.
   ☐ c. lacewing.
   ☐ d. butterfly.

   (15)

2. The aphid lion sheds its skin

   ☐ a. once.
   ☐ b. twice.
   ☐ c. three times.
   ☐ d. four times.

   (15)

3. The writer hints that the aphid lion eats

   ☐ a. unwanted weeds.
   ☐ b. harmful insects.
   ☐ c. flower seeds.
   ☐ d. bacteria.

   (15)

4. Rainbow-tinted wings are

   ☐ a. faint.
   ☐ b. dull.
   ☐ c. drab.
   ☐ d. colorful.

   (15)

5. A good synonym for <u>filament</u> would be

   ☐ a. strand.
   ☐ b. petal.
   ☐ c. shell.
   ☐ d. branch.

   (15)

6. Main Idea

	Answer	Score
Mark the main idea	M	10
Mark the statement that is a detail	D	5
Mark the statement that is too narrow	N	5
Mark the statement that is too broad	B	5

a. The aphid lion's tremendous appetite for aphids causes her to shed her skin several times.

b. The aphid lion can eat aphids for 2 days straight.

c. Some garden insects are natural pest killers.

d. The aphid lion changes into a golden-eyed lacewing about ½ inch (about 1.3 centimeters) long.

Total Comprehension Score
(Add your scores and enter the total on the graph on page 103.)

Categories of Comprehension Questions

No. 1: Subject Matter	No. 4: Clarifying Devices
No. 2: Supporting Details	No. 5: Vocabulary in Context
No. 3: Conclusion	No. 6: Main Idea

20. The Hunter and the Hunted

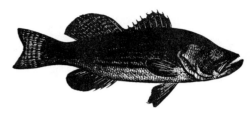
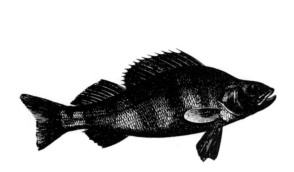

It is the male bass that protects the bass eggs. The eggs hatch three or four days after being laid. Then the tiny bass will head for the dark green grass. Here there is more cover. Each will be about a quarter of an inch (about .64 centimeters) long. They will swarm around their father like bees.

In two or three weeks, the little fry will grow into two-inch (about 5.1 centimeters) *fingerlings*. But out of hundreds hatched, only a few dozen are left. The rest have been eaten by other larger fish.

When the young bass are close to three weeks old, the father will leave them. The fingerlings then scatter to find food. Now on their own, they must learn to watch out for sunfish, pickerel, carp and other bass, even their own parents.

The fingerlings will start eating by nibbling at insect larvae. As they grow, they will become meat-eating hunters in their own right. Their wide mouths will grow wider. They will <u>terrorize</u> the small fish around them. As hunters, they may eat crayfish, snakes, sunfish, bluefish, other small bass and even ducklings and baby muskrats!

A full-grown bass may weigh ten to fifteen pounds (about 4.5 to 6.8 kilograms). A few will grow to twenty-five pounds (about 11.3 kilograms) and measure three feet (about .91 meters) in length. The smartest and strongest of them will go on growing and hunting until they are twenty years old. Some scientists believe they would go on living for many more years. But the bass is always killed. It is taken either by disease or a smarter, faster enemy. An air-breathing mammal from the land, such as the otter, may hunt the water at any time and take the bass for food.

The hunter is now the prey. Yet the life cycle of the bass again repeats itself in the little fry it has left behind.

?

	Possible Score	Your Score

1. This passage is about

   ☐ a. bass.
   ☐ b. pickerel.
   ☐ c. carp.
   ☐ d. sunfish.   15   ○

2. Fingerlings feed on

   ☐ a. fish eggs.
   ☐ b. insect larvae.
   ☐ c. grassy plants.
   ☐ d. algae.   15   ○

3. When a fish first hatches, it is called a

   ☐ a. pup.
   ☐ b. fry.
   ☐ c. fingerling.
   ☐ d. yearling.   15   ○

4. A "full-grown" bass is

   ☐ a. an egg.
   ☐ b. a baby.
   ☐ c. an adult.
   ☐ d. a young female.   15   ○

5. A <u>terrorized</u> fish is

   ☐ a. angry.
   ☐ b. frightened.
   ☐ c. quarrelsome.
   ☐ d. shy.   15   ○

6. Main Idea

	Answer	Score
Mark the main idea	M	10
Mark the statement that is a detail	D	5
Mark the statement that is too narrow	N	5
Mark the statement that is too broad	B	5

a. The life cycle of the bass goes from one extreme to the other.

b. A full-grown bass weighs up to 10 or 15 pounds (about 4.5 – 6.8 kilograms).

c. An adult bass will prey upon crayfish, snakes, sunfish, and bluefish.

d. A young bass starts life hunted by others but grows to be a hunter.

Total Comprehension Score
(Add your scores and enter the total on the graph on page 103.)

Categories of Comprehension Questions

No. 1: Subject Matter	No. 4: Clarifying Devices
No. 2: Supporting Details	No. 5: Vocabulary in Context
No. 3: Conclusion	No. 6: Main Idea

21. The Rattlesnake

There are many different kinds of rattlers in this country, and all of them are poisonous. They do not chase people, but even if they did, you could out-walk the fastest rattler.

Not all rattlesnakes behave the same way. Some rattlers wind themselves into a high coil and just look very fierce. Others will rattle a warning the moment they see you. A few will strike without making a sound. The timid ones wait silently, as though hoping you won't notice them. Still others slither backward to escape. Then there are rattlers that hiss at you without rattling at all.

Rattlesnakes do have one thing in common. They have two pits, one on each side of the face. This is why they are called *pit vipers*.

Some people believe that a rattler is helpless just before it sheds its skin. This is not so, for even though the snake is "milky-eyed" and its vision is blurry at this time, its facial pits can sense heat. The rattlesnake can always detect anything that is warmer than the surrounding air, such as a mouse, a rabbit or a human hand or foot and will strike at it.

A newborn rattler has a "button" on the tip of its tail, but it can't make a rattling sound until it is about ten days old. At that time the skin is shed and the first "rattle" appears. Each time the snake sheds its skin a new rattle will appear. This usually happens two or three times every year.

Do not be afraid of the rattler's forked tongue when it darts out. The tongue is the snake's organ of touch and smell and is actually harmless. It is the rattler's fangs that are dangerous. Rattlers are born with fangs which are needle-like, hollow teeth. These fangs inject the deadly poison, or *venom,* into their victims.

Usually the fangs are folded back in the top of the rattler's mouth. When the snake strikes, its mouth opens and the fangs are projected forward. As the snake bites its prey, the poison flows out of the fangs into the victim. This is the rattlesnake's only way of killing the animals and birds upon which it feeds. However, it will also bite to defend itself.

Young rattlers, which can strike even more quickly than mature snakes, are also deadly because they are born with a full supply of venom. So beware of the youngsters; they are dangerous too!

Don't panic if you see a rattlesnake, but be sure to keep your distance. They can't jump through the air at you. They can strike only the distance of their own length. Be careful anyway and have respect for rattlers.

?

	Possible Score	Your Score

1. What would be another good title for this passage?

    ☐ a. Timber Rattlers
    ☐ b. A Rattlesnake Farm
    ☐ c. The Helpless Rattler
    ☐ d. All about Rattlesnakes

    (15)

2. The rattlesnake uses its tongue

    ☐ a. to smell.
    ☐ b. to bite.
    ☐ c. to hear.
    ☐ d. to inject poison.

    (15)

3. A rattlesnake cannot make a rattling sound until it

    ☐ a. loses its fangs.
    ☐ b. attacks its first victim.
    ☐ c. sheds its first skin.
    ☐ d. spends one winter hibernating.

    (15)

4. The second paragraph tells us that some rattlesnakes are

    ☐ a. pit vipers.
    ☐ b. not deadly.
    ☐ c. milky-eyed.
    ☐ d. shy.

    (15)

5. Facial pits are located on the snake's

    ☐ a. tail.
    ☐ b. face.
    ☐ c. stomach.
    ☐ d. back.

    (15)

6. Main Idea

	Answer	Score
Mark the main idea	M	10
Mark the statement that is a detail	D	5
Mark the statement that is too narrow	N	5
Mark the statement that is too broad	B	5

a. Rattlesnakes will bite to inject deadly venom.

b. Each time a rattler sheds its skin, a new rattle will appear.

c. All rattlesnakes have rattles and fangs which inject poison.

d. Some snakes are dangerous to humans.

Total Comprehension Score
(Add your scores and enter the total on the graph on page 103.)

Categories of Comprehension Questions

No. 1: Subject Matter	No. 4: Clarifying Devices
No. 2: Supporting Details	No. 5: Vocabulary in Context
No. 3: Conclusion	No. 6: Main Idea

22. The Hungry Sea Anemone

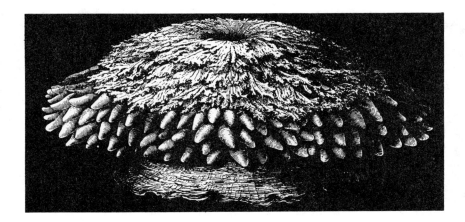

I once saw a hungry sea anemone (a NEM o ne) catch a small white clam. It used its two rows of tentacles around the edge of its mouth to grab the clam. In a few minutes the mouth covered the whole clam. At the same time, the anemone's muscles pulled the clam into its body where it could be digested.

About twenty minutes later the anemone slowly pushed out the empty clamshell. It had <u>digested</u> the soft flesh of the clam. Now it threw out what it did not want.

If you ever search along a rocky coast, you might see sea anemones clinging to the rocks under the water. At first glance you might think they are a type of flower, but these creatures are animals.

There are about 1,000 kinds of sea anemones. Many live in *tide pools*. These are the pools of water left among rocks when the tide goes out. These anemones depend on the ebb and flow of the water to bring them food. They eat clams and such things as small fish, crabs and plankton.

They never seem to stop eating. As each wave comes in, it brings food with it. The anemones wave their tentacles through the water. Those that eat larger prey paralyze it with the stinging cells on their tentacles. Then they push the prey into their mouths. The smaller anemones use their tentacles to "sweep" plankton from the water and into their mouths.

As the tide goes out, the anemones that are attached to rocks or wharfs above the water grow still. They close up, each looking like a small, round ball, with just their mouths showing.

Some anemones can move and search for a place to live. They may slide on their foot pad. Or they may let go and float. Some can walk upside down on their tentacles until they find just the right spot.

?
_____

	Possible Score	Your Score

1. The sea anemone is

    ☐ a. an animal.
    ☐ b. a plant.
    ☐ c. a mollusk.
    ☐ d. seaweed.

    (15)   ◯

2. How many kinds of anemones are there?

    ☐ a. 10
    ☐ b. 200
    ☐ c. 500
    ☐ d. 1,000

    (15)   ◯

3. In order to eat, the anemone must depend upon

    ☐ a. other fish to feed it.
    ☐ b. large amounts of seaweed.
    ☐ c. the food dropped by seagulls.
    ☐ d. the tide to bring it food.

    (15)   ◯

4. The ebb and flow of the water refers to

    ☐ a. the amount of salt in the ocean.
    ☐ b. the tide.
    ☐ c. the strength of the waves.
    ☐ d. the amount of bacteria in the water.

    (15)   ◯

5. The anemone <u>digested</u> the clam. This means the anemone

    ☐ a. ate the clam.
    ☐ b. fought the clam.
    ☐ c. captured the clam.
    ☐ d. found the clam.

    (15)   ◯

6. Main Idea

	Answer	Score
Mark the main idea	M	10
Mark the statement that is a detail	D	5
Mark the statement that is too narrow	N	5
Mark the statement that is too broad	B	5

a. Some sea anemones can eat a whole clam at once.

b. Sea anemones spend most of their time eating.

c. Sea anemones are animals, but look like flowers.

d. Some animals have tremendous appetites.

Total Comprehension Score
(Add your scores and enter the total on the graph on page 103.)

Categories of Comprehension Questions

No. 1: Subject Matter	No. 4: Clarifying Devices
No. 2: Supporting Details	No. 5: Vocabulary in Context
No. 3: Conclusion	No. 6: Main Idea

23. Jaguar

Onca the jaguar was hungry. Her last meal had been eaten five days earlier when her mother had killed a *capybara*, the largest of all rodents. Now her mother was gone; her brother was gone. Onca was hungry and alone in the Brazilian rain forest.

Onca was on her own. When hunger first gripped her, she tried to catch fish as her mother had. But she was still clumsy, and the fish got away. She charged a group of peccaries, but they scattered. She almost got a brocket deer, called *corzuela* (kor ZOO ee lah) by the natives. But another hunter, a puma, beat her to the kill. Pumas and jaguars are the two species of great cats found in the western hemisphere.

The puma which Onca met weighed only eighty pounds (about 36.3 kilograms). Onca weighed almost one hundred (about 45.4 kilograms). But the puma was faster than Onca and drove her away from the deer. It was older and experienced; Onca was no match for it.

Late in the afternoon, the jaguar walked to the river to drink. The sun's rays glistened on her thick, yellow coat with its dark brown rosettes. Onca looked very much like her African relative, the leopard.

As Onca crouched drinking at the river, she heard the sound of a twig snap. Slowly, quietly, she backed into the bushes and waited. Maybe this would be food. Sure enough, a small capybara came along. Onca waited. Her earlier mistake in charging the peccaries too soon had taught her patience. When the capybara was within ten feet (about 3.1 meters), the jaguar attacked. She knocked the capybara down, but she had not yet learned how to make a fast kill. The capybara dragged her into the river. But Onca was almost as much at home there as on dry land. She held on and the fight soon ended in death for the capybara. Onca dragged the carcass out of the water and, for the first time in five days, she ate. Afterward, she buried what was left for later meals.

Now the past with mother and brother was truly gone. With this kill, Onca had proved she could take care of herself. She would make many more kills in the years to come. Her worst enemy would be people. If she were lucky, she could avoid people, and, if she didn't become sick or crippled, she might live to be twenty years old.

That would come in its time. For now, her belly was full. Onca the jaguar rose and walked slowly into her home, the <u>tropical</u> <u>rain</u> <u>forest</u>.

?

	Possible Score	Your Score

1. This passage is about

    ☐ a. pumas and jaguars.
    ☐ b. hunting a jaguar.
    ☐ c. the parents of a jaguar.
    ☐ d. a young jaguar.

    (15)

2. Pumas and jaguars are found in the

    ☐ a. northern hemisphere.
    ☐ b. southern hemisphere.
    ☐ c. eastern hemisphere.
    ☐ d. western hemisphere.

    (15)

3. It seems that a puma

    ☐ a. is smaller than a jaguar.
    ☐ b. is exactly like a jaguar.
    ☐ c. is much larger than a jaguar.
    ☐ d. has much nicer fur than a jaguar.

    (15)

4. As Onca quietly waited in the bushes, she showed that jaguars can be very

    ☐ a. tense.
    ☐ b. patient.
    ☐ c. careless.
    ☐ d. nervous.

    (15)

5. A <u>tropical</u> <u>rain</u> <u>forest</u> is a

    ☐ a. butte.
    ☐ b. plateau.
    ☐ c. thicket.
    ☐ d. jungle.

    (15)

6. Main Idea

	Answer	Score
Mark the main idea	M	10
Mark the statement that is a detail	D	5
Mark the statement that is too narrow	N	5
Mark the statement that is too broad	B	5

a. Onca the jaguar killed a small capybara.

b. Onca the jaguar learned how to hunt.

c. Jaguars have yellow coats with dark brown rosettes.

d. Jaguars are skilled hunters.

Total Comprehension Score
(Add your scores and enter the
total on the graph on page 103.)

Categories of Comprehension Questions

No. 1: Subject Matter	No. 4: Clarifying Devices
No. 2: Supporting Details	No. 5: Vocabulary in Context
No. 3: Conclusion	No. 6: Main Idea

24. Quilting Get-Togethers

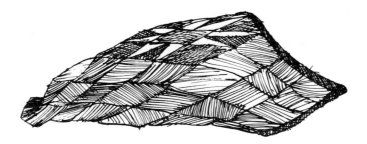

In the 1800s farm folks knew three kinds of bees: the winged bees for honey, the barn-raising bees for men, and the quilting bees for women.

The golden age of quilt-making was from the early 1800s until about 1880. A woman was asked to go to many sewing bees. If her stitches were very small, she would be given a place to work around the frame. Poor needle-workers might be edged quietly toward the kitchen. Here they would help with the turkey.

The first quilts, or bedspreads, were not often beautiful. Cloth was hard to get in those early days. Each piece had to be brought from far off lands or made by hand at home. Clothes were worn, then made over and used again. If there was any good cloth left, it was used in making a warm cover for the bed.

Quilting get-togethers <u>bridged</u> the long distance between houses. They were happy breaks in days of hard work. Women wore their Sunday best and arrived early in the morning. The guests quilted swiftly and steadily. They laughed and talked as they worked. At a bee, all the neighborhood turned out. One group of women would work for a while; then another group would take over.

Such a party always ended with a big meal to which the men came. The evening flew by, with singing, dancing and games.

?

	Possible Score	Your Score

1. This passage talks mostly about

   ☐ a. how quilting bees first began.
   ☐ b. the kinds of cloth used for quilt-making.
   ☐ c. quilting as a reason for getting together.
   ☐ d. how members of a quilting bee were chosen.

   (15)

2. How long was the golden age of quilt making?

   ☐ a. 50 years
   ☐ b. 80 years
   ☐ c. 100 years
   ☐ d. 200 years

   (15)

3. Why were quilting bees so popular?

   ☐ a. They gave people a chance to visit.
   ☐ b. The best quilts were made at bees.
   ☐ c. They were more fun than barn-raising bees.
   ☐ d. Bedspreads were too hard to make alone.

   (15)

4. The first paragraph was meant to be a joke. Why?

   ☐ a. People had fun at quilting bees.
   ☐ b. Barn-raising stories are always funny.
   ☐ c. Men also went to quilting bees.
   ☐ d. The word "bees" has two meanings.

   (15)

5. When long distances are <u>bridged</u>, people

   ☐ a. become farther apart.
   ☐ b. attend more parties.
   ☐ c. become closer together.
   ☐ d. stay home more.

   (15)

6. Main Idea

	Answer	Score
Mark the main idea	M	10
Mark the statement that is a detail	D	5
Mark the statement that is too narrow	N	5
Mark the statement that is too broad	B	5

a. Quilt-making in the 1800s was an enjoyable social event.

b. The 1840s farm folk held two kinds of "bees."

c. The finest quilts were made with very small stitches.

d. The guests quilted swiftly and steadily.

Total Comprehension Score
(Add your scores and enter the
total on the graph on page 103.)

Categories of Comprehension Questions

No. 1: Subject Matter	No. 4: Clarifying Devices
No. 2: Supporting Details	No. 5: Vocabulary in Context
No. 3: Conclusion	No. 6: Main Idea

25. When Winter Comes

Many kinds of animals stay active year-round. Trout, pike and other cold-water fish go through the winter with hardly any changes. But other animals must prepare for the cold. Deer, grouse and other warm-blooded animals build up layers of fat on their bodies. Squirrels store nuts. Beavers stick twigs and branches into the mud at the bottom of their pond. These will provide snacks all through the winter. Pikas, small rabbits of the western mountains, store food piles of dried grass.

Other animals change their diets. Cardinals give up their insect diet and eat mostly seeds. Cottontail rabbits nibble twigs instead of juicy leaves.

Many mammals grow an extra coat of fur which protects them from the cold. Deer grow extra, hollow hairs which do a great job of keeping them warm. Musk oxen grow a long shaggy coat of hair over their soft undercoat. The long hair protects them from rain and snow, and the undercoat helps to hold in body heat.

Birds keep in their body heat by fluffing out their feathers to make a thicker coat. Ducks and geese have undercoats of soft down. Bobwhite quail sleep at night snuggled up in a tight, cozy circle.

Some animals survive winter by leaving the cold country — they migrate. Some make very short trips. Mountain quail walk downhill in single file to warmer valleys where they spend the winter. Certain fish, such as bluefish, migrate short distances to warmer water.

Other animals migrate only about 100 miles (about 161 kilometers). Caribou of the Arctic move south from the tundra to find food and shelter in the forests. Canadian geese fly south until they find water that doesn't freeze over and fields that are not snow covered all winter. Bluebirds fly south until they find places where there is plenty of food. Dragonflies, which are the strongest of all flying insects, migrate ahead of winter. Deer and mountain sheep move down from high mountain summer ranges to warmer winter pastures on lower ground.

Some animals migrate great distances. Arctic terns fly 11,000 miles (about 17,710 kilometers) from the Arctic to the tip of South America. And monarch butterflies fly several hundred miles south.

Winter means long months of hardship for many animals. But one day a warm breeze blows from the south. Soon streams run full with melting snow and ice. Trees burst into bloom. And then, suddenly it seems, spring arrives. Robins return and sing their cheery songs. Moths <u>stir</u> in their cocoons. Frogs crawl from the mud. Groundhogs poke their sleepy heads from their burrows. Soon animal babies will be born. The wild creatures have survived another winter.

?

| | Possible Score | Your Score |

1. What would be another good title for this passage?

   ☐ a. Nature's Hibernating Creatures
   ☐ b. Trees in Winter
   ☐ c. Preparing for Winter
   ☐ d. That Winter White Stuff

   (15)   ◯

2. The strongest of all flying insects is the

   ☐ a. spider.
   ☐ b. housefly.
   ☐ c. mosquito.
   ☐ d. dragonfly.

   (15)   ◯

3. The writer hints that one of the dangers of winter is the lack of

   ☐ a. hibernation.
   ☐ b. food.
   ☐ c. snow.
   ☐ d. sunshine.

   (15)   ◯

4. A robin's cheery song would sound

   ☐ a. soft and sad.
   ☐ b. weak and low.
   ☐ c. lively and happy.
   ☐ d. nervous and loud.

   (15)   ◯

5. As used in this passage, stir means

   ☐ a. to move.
   ☐ b. to eat.
   ☐ c. to sleep.
   ☐ d. to fly.

   (15)   ◯

6. Main Idea

	Answer	Score
Mark the main idea	M	10
Mark the statement that is a detail	D	5
Mark the statement that is too narrow	N	5
Mark the statement that is too broad	B	5

a. Robins return in the spring to sing their songs.

b. Animals survive the winter in many ways.

c. Birds keep in their body heat by fluffing out their feathers to make a thicker covering.

d. Living creatures which stay active all winter survive the cold in different ways.

Total Comprehension Score
(Add your scores and enter the total on the graph on page 103.)

Categories of Comprehension Questions

No. 1: Subject Matter	No. 4: Clarifying Devices
No. 2: Supporting Details	No. 5: Vocabulary in Context
No. 3: Conclusion	No. 6: Main Idea

Acknowledgments

The passages appearing in this book have been reprinted with the kind permission of the following publications and publishers to whom the author is indebted:

Aramco World Magazine, published by The Arabian American Oil Company, New York, New York.

The Communicator, published by the New York State Outdoor Education Association, Syracuse, New York.

The Conservationist, published by the New York State Conservation Department, Albany, New York.

A Cornell Science Leaflet, published by the New York State College of Agriculture and Life Sciences, a unit of the State University, at Cornell University, Ithaca, New York.

Food, The Yearbook of Agriculture, published by the United States Department of Agriculture, Washington, D.C.

Handbook of Nature-Study, published by Comstock Publishing Company, Ithaca, New York.

Kansas Fish & Game, published by the Kansas Forestry, Fish and Game Commission, Pratt, Kansas.

National Wildlife, published by The National Wildlife Federation, Washington, D.C.

Outdoor Oklahoma, published by the Oklahoma Department of Wildlife Conservation, Oklahoma City, Oklahoma.

Pennsylvania Game News, published by the Pennsylvania Game Commission, Harrisburg, Pennsylvania.

Ranger Rick's Nature Magazine, published by The National Wildlife Federation, Washington, D.C.

The Tennessee Conservationist, published by the Tennessee Department of Conservation and the Tennessee Game and Fish Commission.

Answer Key: Book 6

Passage 1:	1.a	2.b	3.b	4.c	5.c	6a.D	6b.M	6c.N	6d.B
Passage 2:	1.d	2.b	3.d	4.a	5.b	6a.D	6b.B	6c.M	6d.N
Passage 3:	1.c	2.d	3.b	4.b	5.c	6a.M	6b.N	6c.D	6d.B
Passage 4:	1.d	2.b	3.c	4.a	5.c	6a.N	6b.B	6c.M	6d.D
Passage 5:	1.c	2.d	3.b	4.c	5.d	6a.M	6b.D	6c.B	6d.N
Passage 6:	1.d	2.a	3.c	4.d	5.b	6a.D	6b.M	6c.B	6d.N
Passage 7:	1.b	2.c	3.b	4.a	5.d	6a.M	6b.B	6c.N	6d.D
Passage 8:	1.b	2.c	3.d	4.a	5.b	6a.M	6b.D	6c.B	6d.N
Passage 9:	1.a	2.d	3.c	4.a	5.b	6a.B	6b.D	6c.N	6d.M
Passage 10:	1.d	2.a	3.b	4.b	5.d	6a.D	6b.M	6c.B	6d.N
Passage 11:	1.b	2.d	3.a	4.c	5.d	6a.B	6b.N	6c.M	6d.D
Passage 12:	1.c	2.b	3.a	4.c	5.d	6a.D	6b.B	6c.N	6d.M

Answer Key: Book 6

Passage 13:	1.c	2.b	3.d	4.b	5.d	6a.B	6b.M	6c.N	6d.D
Passage 14:	1.c	2.c	3.a	4.b	5.d	6a.D	6b.M	6c.N	6d.B
Passage 15:	1.a	2.d	3.b	4.b	5.c	6a.N	6b.B	6c.D	6d.M
Passage 16:	1.d	2.a	3.c	4.d	5.c	6a.B	6b.N	6c.D	6d.M
Passage 17:	1.d	2.b	3.d	4.a	5.c	6a.D	6b.B	6c.N	6d.M
Passage 18:	1.b	2.a	3.c	4.d	5.c	6a.B	6b.N	6c.M	6d.D
Passage 19:	1.c	2.d	3.b	4.d	5.a	6a.M	6b.N	6c.B	6d.D
Passage 20:	1.a	2.b	3.b	4.c	5.b	6a.B	6b.D	6c.N	6d.M
Passage 21:	1.d	2.a	3.c	4.d	5.b	6a.N	6b.D	6c.M	6d.B
Passage 22:	1.a	2.d	3.d	4.b	5.a	6a.N	6b.M	6c.D	6d.B
Passage 23:	1.d	2.d	3.a	4.b	5.d	6a.N	6b.M	6c.D	6d.B
Passage 24:	1.c	2.b	3.a	4.d	5.c	6a.M	6b.B	6c.N	6d.D
Passage 25:	1.c	2.d	3.b	4.c	5.a	6a.D	6b.B	6c.N	6d.M

Diagnostic Chart (For Student Correction)

Directions: Write your final answers in the *upper* part of the passage block. Then correct your answers using the Answer Key on pages 100 and 101. If your answer is correct, do not make any more marks in the block. If your answer is incorrect, write the letter of the correct answer in the *lower* part of the block.

Categories of Comprehension Skills	Reading Passage 1-25
1. Subject Matter	
2. Supporting Details	
3. Conclusion	
4. Clarifying Devices	
5. Vocabulary in Context	
6. Main Idea — Main Idea	
Detail	
Too Narrow	
Too Broad	

Progress Graph

Directions: Write your Total Comprehension Score in the box under the number for each passage. Then put an *x* along the line above each box to show your Total Comprehension Score for that passage. Then make a graph of your progress. Draw a line to connect the *x*'s.

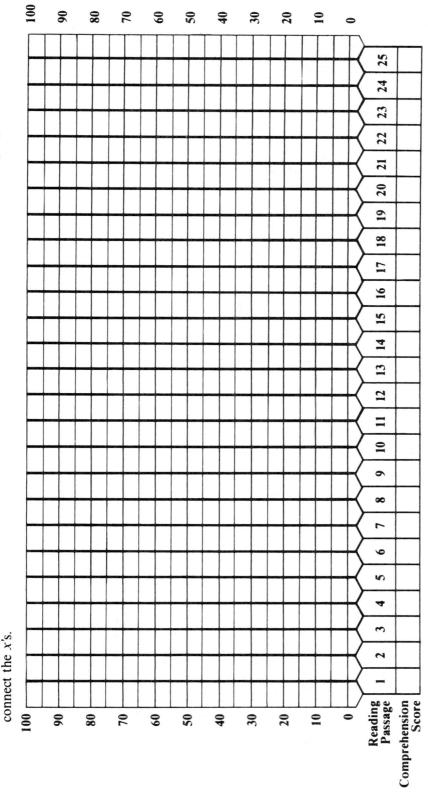

Classroom Management System

Essential Skills Series

Classroom Management System
(For Teacher Correction)

To the Teacher

The Classroom Management System provides an easy and effective way to individualize instruction. It can be used by reading specialists as well as by regular classroom teachers. The management system is designed to be equally effective when used with a single student, a small group, or a full-size class.

The Classroom Management System provides ongoing assessment of student work for both you and your student. It shows not only the amount of work completed, but also the quality of the work.

It serves as a diagnostic tool by revealing patterns of errors at a glance. For example, if a student has difficulty identifying subject matter (question #1 in each set of questions throughout the *Essential Skills Series*), a pattern of errors will appear in the Subject Matter column of the Classroom Management System Record Sheet. This will enable you to focus on the specific skills needs of each student.

The Classroom Management System Record Sheet is on pages 108-109. Both pages may be duplicated and stapled together.

How to Use the Classroom Management System Record Sheet

Step 1: Have the student answer the questions for each *Essential Skills* passage under the appropriate question heading.

Passage	① Subject Matter	② Supporting Details	③ Conclusion	④ Clarifying Devices	⑤ Vocabulary in Context	⑥ Main Idea a b c d	Number Correct	Errors Corrected
1	a	c	a	b	d	N D B M		

Step 2: Circle any incorrect answers and fill in the total number correct.

| 1 | a | ⓒ | a | b | d | Ⓝ D B M | 6 | |

Step 3: Have the student correct his or her incorrect answers.

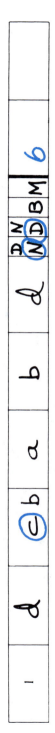

Step 4: Give assistance as needed and, if necessary, correct the student's adjusted answers.

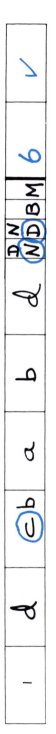

Step 5: Have the student go on to the next passage.

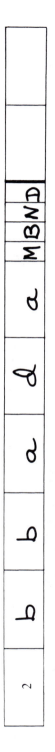

Step 6: Repeat Steps 1-4. If the class is large, it may be necessary to have students complete two or three passages before you correct them. This will slow the "traffic" at your desk.

Note: It is important for students to analyze and, to the extent possible, correct their own errors (Step 3).

Essential Skills Series

Classroom Management System Record Sheet
(For Teacher Correction)

Name _____

Teacher _____

Date _____

Book Number _____

To the Student: Write your answers in the spaces provided. (See the Example below.) Your teacher will circle any incorrect answers. Then go back over the questions and correct your mistakes.

Passage	① Subject Matter	② Supporting Details	③ Conclusion	④ Clarifying Devices	⑤ Vocabulary in Context	⑥ Main Idea a b c d	Number Correct	Errors Corrected
Example	c	(b) a	d	a	c	a (b) c d / a (b) M B		
1								
2								
3								
4								
5								
6								
7								
8								
9								
10								

	①	②	③	④	⑤	⑥
11						
12						
13						
14						
15						
16						
17						
18						
19						
20						
21						
22						
23						
24						
25						

This record sheet may be duplicated for classroom use by teachers. From *Essential Skills Series* by Walter Pauk, copyright © 1982 by Jamestown Publishers. Classroom Management System by Thomas F. Kelly, Ph.D.